How to Quickly and Accurately Master Arrhythmia Interpretation

DALE DAVIS, RCT
Montville, New Jersey

Illustrated by Patrick Turner

J. B. LIPPINCOTT COMPANY Philadelphia
London Mexico City New York
St. Louis São Paulo Sydney

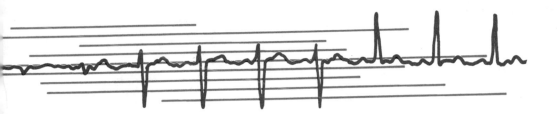

*How to Quickly and
Accurately Master*

ARRHYTHMIA

Interpretation

Acquisitions Editor: Charles McCormick
Manuscript Editor: Lee Henderson
Indexer: Ann Cassar
Design Coordinator: Caren Erlichman
Designer: Anne O'Donnell
Production Manager: Carol A. Florence
Production Coordinator: Barney Fernandes
Compositor: Bi-Comp, Inc.
Printer/Binder: R. R. Donnelley & Sons Company
Cover Printer: Lehigh Press

6 5 4 3 2 1

Library of Congress Cataloging-in-Publication Data

Davis, Dale.
  How to quickly and accurately master arrhythmia
interpretation.

    Includes index.
    1. Arrhythmia—Diagnosis. 2. Electrocardiography—
Interpretation. I. Title. [DNLM: 1. Arrhythmias—
diagnosis—programmed instruction. 2. Electro-
cardiography—programmed instruction. WG 18 D2609h]
RC685.A65D38 1989   616.1'280754   88-6819
ISBN 0-397-50947-2

PREFACE

Paramedics and critical care and intensive care monitoring personnel need to learn arrhythmia interpretation, but they must also develop the ability to make quick and accurate interpretations without the assistance of calipers, careful classroom measurements, and perfect ECG strips.

Until now, this skill had to be learned on the job, over long periods, and with substantial numbers of ECG strips for practice. But now, with *How to Quickly and Accurately Master Arrhythmia Interpretation*, an arrhythmia book geared for emergency monitoring personnel, this vital skill can be acquired with the use of simplified criteria geared for quick and accurate "eyeball" interpretations and can then be honed to perfection by interpreting the practice strips at the end of each chapter.

The book is simply organized and includes easy-to-understand diagrams that enhance the text and ensure comprehension rather than just memorization of criteria. I have intentionally chosen simplicity over exactness in some areas of the book to make learning uncomplicated.

In Chapters 1 through 12, each arrhythmia is presented with a diagram of the electrical conduction system and an explanation of the electrophysiology of the respective arrhythmia, a simplified list of criteria for rapid and accurate interpretation, and a number of ECG strips representing the arrhythmia, labeled not only with the interpretation but also with the exact criteria and step-by-step method used to arrive at the solution. Dozens of practice strips interspersed throughout the book allow the student to obtain the necessary skills to become proficient in rapid and accurate emergency arrhythmia detection.

Chapter 13 is a unique chapter in that it takes you from the initial impressions of the strip through a step-by-step process to the final interpretation and instructs and drills you in the art of "eyeballing" an interpretation. It enables you to become proficient at the skills of quickness and accuracy in interpretation in a short period and to become accustomed to less-than-perfect ECG monitoring strips.

This book is directed toward those in the allied health, nursing, or medical fields who desire to master arrhythmia interpretation and at the same time understand the electrophysiology of arrhythmias and be able to rapidly and accurately identify them without the use of calipers, rate rulers, and careful classroom measurements.

Dale Davis, RCT

ACKNOWLEDGMENTS

I want to thank Barbara Bell and Donna Dicksheid of the Cardiac Services Department of Morristown Memorial Hospital, Morristown, NJ, for their help in collecting arrhythmia tracings.

Many thanks to my illustrator, Patrick Turner, for his creativity and for his patience with my often confusing instructions.

I am grateful to my publisher, J. B. Lippincott Company, for allowing me great freedom both in the layout of this book and in the reproduction of the ECG strips in color. My thanks to Lisa A. Biello for her enthusiasm and for the encouragement she has given me with this book and its predecessor.

CONTENTS

1 ONE-LEAD MONITORING *1*
Lead Placement *2*
Standard Leads *4*
Artifact *6*

2 ELECTROPHYSIOLOGY AND THE ELECTRICAL CONDUCTION SYSTEM *9*
Depolarization and Repolarization *10*
Anatomy *11*
The Electrical Conduction System *13*
Intervals and Segments *20*

3 ECG GRAPH PAPER AND MEASUREMENTS *21*
Time and Voltage *22*
Measurements *25*
Practice ECG Strips *29*
Practice ECG Strip Answers *33*

4 DETERMINATION OF HEART RATE AND SINUS RHYTHMS *35*
Determination of Heart Rate *36*
Sinus Rhythms *37*
Practice ECG Strips *46*
Practice ECG Strip Answers *52*

5 PREMATURE CONTRACTIONS *53*
Atrial Premature Contraction *54*
AV Nodal or Junctional Premature Contraction *59*
Ventricular Premature Contraction *62*
Differential Diagnosis *68*
Practice ECG Strips *71*
Practice ECG Strip Answers *77*

6 ESCAPE BEATS AND RHYTHMS   79
   Junctional Escape Beat   80
   Junctional Escape Rhythm   83
   Ventricular Escape Beat   84
   Ventricular Escape Rhythm   86
   Differential Diagnosis   87
   Practice ECG Strips   89
   Practice ECG Strip Answers   95

7 SUPRAVENTRICULAR ECTOPIC RHYTHMS   97
   Atrial Rhythms   98
   Junctional Rhythms   115
   Supraventricular Tachycardia   120
   Differential Diagnosis   121
   Practice ECG Strips   125
   Practice ECG Strip Answers   133

8 VENTRICULAR ECTOPIC RHYTHMS   135
   Accelerated Idioventricular Rhythm   136
   Ventricular Tachycardia   138
   Ventricular Flutter   141
   Ventricular Fibrillation   143
   Differential Diagnosis   145
   Practice ECG Strips   150
   Practice ECG Strip Answers   156

9 ABERRATION AND WOLFF–PARKINSON–WHITE SYNDROME   157
   Aberration   158
   Wolff–Parkinson–White Syndrome   164
   Differential Diagnosis   167
   Practice ECG Strips   170
   Practice ECG Strip Answers   176

10 AV BLOCK   177
   First Degree AV Block   178
   Second Degree AV Block Wenckebach   178
   Second Degree AV Block Mobitz   181
   High Grade AV Block   184
   Complete AV Block   187
   Differential Diagnosis   191
   Practice ECG Strips   195
   Practice ECG Strip Answers   201

CONTENTS

x

11 SA BLOCK *203*
First Degree SA Block *204*
Second Degree SA Block *204*
Differential Diagnosis *208*
Practice ECG Strips *211*
Practice ECG Strip Answers *217*

12 PACEMAKER RHYTHMS *219*
Normal Pacemaker Function *220*
Pacemaker Malfunction *224*
Differential Diagnosis *228*
Practice ECG Strips *231*
Practice ECG Strip Answers *237*

13 HOW TO MAKE RAPID AND ACCURATE INTERPRETATIONS IN THE FIELD *239*

INDEX *271*

CONTENTS

How to Quickly and Accurately Master Arrhythmia Interpretation

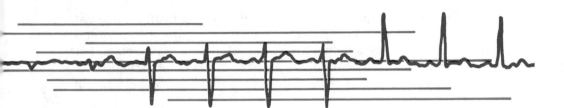

Chapter 1

ONE-LEAD MONITORING

An electrocardiogram (ECG) is a recording of the heart's electrical activity as viewed from 12 different positions around the heart. It enables one to make certain assumptions about the condition and size of the heart muscle, to interpret the rhythm of the heart, and to note any abnormal heartbeats or rhythms (arrhythmias) that are present.

One-lead monitoring records the heart's electrical activity as viewed from only one position around the heart. One can ascertain rhythms and diagnose arrhythmias from one-lead monitoring, but one cannot make assumptions about the condition or size of the heart muscle.

LEAD PLACEMENT

Electrodes are placed on the patient's wrists and left leg, or they may be placed on the upper and lower torso, one by each shoulder and the remaining one at the bottom of the left side of the rib cage. A fourth electrode is placed on the right ankle or right lower rib cage to stabilize the ECG, but this fourth electrode takes no part in lead formation. Other electrode placements can be used at your discretion.

Ideal electrode placement should be on clean, dry areas of skin, as free of hair and surface imperfections as possible. Because muscle movement creates artifact, the ECG recording will be of better quality if the electrodes are placed over bone rather than muscle and if the patient remains as nearly immobile as possible.

ELECTRODE PLACEMENT ON LIMBS

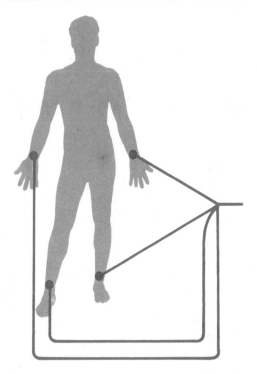

ELECTRODE PLACEMENT ON TORSO

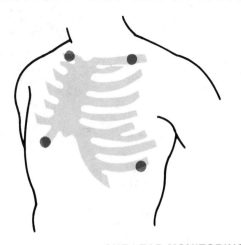

ONE-LEAD MONITORING

STANDARD LEADS

Standard leads are commonly used in one-lead monitoring. They are called bipolar leads because they are composed of two electrodes—one negative and one positive—and the monitoring machine records the difference in electrical potential between them. Although you can usually view only one lead at a time during emergency monitoring, you can often view three different leads individually.

Lead I is composed of the right arm, which is designated a negative electrode, and the left arm, which is considered a positive electrode.

LEAD I

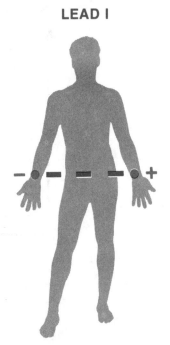

LEAD II

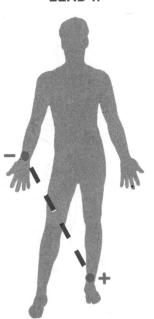

Lead II is composed of the right arm, considered the negative electrode, and the left leg, designated the positive electrode.

Lead III is composed of the left arm, considered the negative electrode, and the left leg, designated the positive electrode.

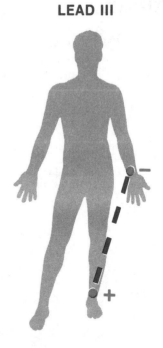

When scanning an entire ECG for an analysis of the heart rhythm, one has the luxury of looking at the heart's electrical activity from 12 different angles or leads to make a rhythm diagnosis. The patient is usually resting and motionless on a bed or examination table, and this makes the ECG free of any outside interference or artifact. However, with one-lead monitoring, used in emergencies, during holter monitoring, or during monitoring in a cardiac or intensive care ward, only one lead is available to make the same rhythm diagnosis. The patient is rarely immobile and is often unable to remain still, leading to less-than-perfect ECG strips often filled with artifact.

So with less information than an ECG provides—and even *this* information is often inferior—the same accurate diagnosis of the heart rhythm must be made from a one-lead ECG strip. The monitoring situation demands quick and accurate interpretations because of life-threatening heart rhythms that often occur.

ARTIFACT

Any outside interference that causes marks on the ECG strip other than the electrical activity of the heart is called *artifact*. It makes quick and accurate arrhythmia identification difficult or impossible. During routine ECG recordings the patient is usually extremely cooperative and can be placed on a comfortable bed with a pillow and can be requested to remain perfectly still for a short period. Portable or bedside monitoring is not ideal for perfect ECG tracings. Monitoring usually occurs over longer periods than an average 1- to 5-minute ECG, and the patient is rarely entirely still and relaxed. The patient may be unconscious or uncooperative, or he may be being monitored over a long period, during which inactivity is impossible.

An ECG tracing begins with a thin horizontal line called a *baseline* or *isoelectric line*, which is recorded on ECG graph paper as the paper moves through the recording machine at 25 mm/second. The electrical activity of the heart is recorded either above or below this line. Artifact that occurs either thickens or distorts the baseline and/or the markings representing electrical activity of the heart and often makes arrhythmia identification difficult or impossible.

AC Interference

Originates from electrical interference at the patient's bedside and causes a thick baseline on the ECG. It could arise directly from metal objects surrounding the patient or from nearby electrical equipment. If time is available, one might disconnect unnecessary and adjacent electrical equipment.

AC INTERFERENCE

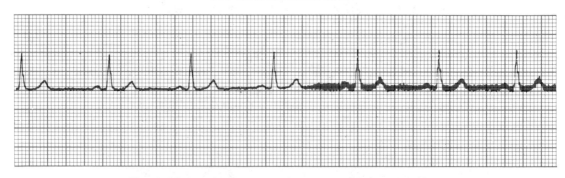

The initial portion of the ECG strip shows no artifact, but the latter portion demonstrates the thickened and darkened tracing present with AC interference.

Muscle Tremor or Patient Movement Artifact

Is generated by the patient himself. It can range from mild to absolutely unacceptable. Placing the electrodes over bone on the torso or limbs often helps if the patient is immobile and only his muscles are tense. If the patient is moving, it is only hoped that a tracing can be run during a quieter moment.

MUSCLE TREMOR

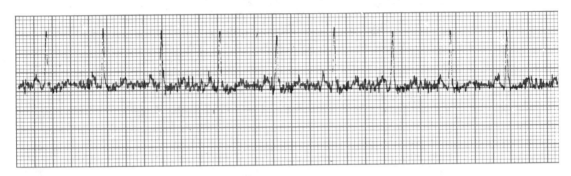

PATIENT MOVEMENT

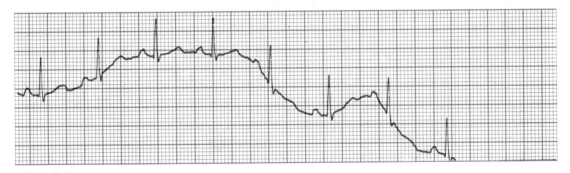

Wandering Baseline

Is often caused by poor electrode contact with the patient's skin. Good contact can be inhibited by excess body hair or by oily, dirty, scaly, or moist skin. Reapplying new electrodes to a better area of the skin may improve the situation, but usually the poor tracing remains, and identification is again made difficult by artifact superimposed on the ECG tracing. Diaphoresis (profuse sweating), often accompanying acute myocardial infarction, makes ECG monitoring extremely difficult because electrode contact is very poor. Attempting to dry the skin where electrodes are placed and then reattaching fresh electrodes may solve very short term monitoring problems, but artifact often returns as electrode contact again becomes poorer.

WANDERING BASELINE

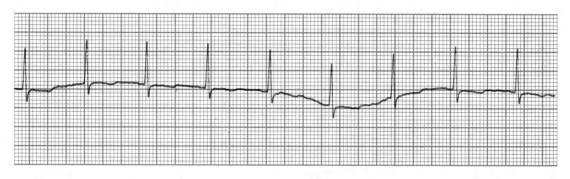

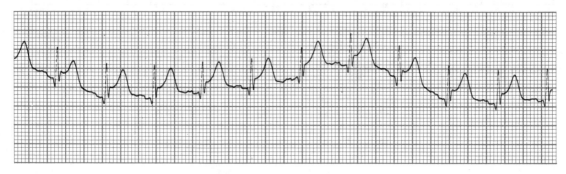

Wandering baseline on an ECG taken during an acute myocardial infarction. The patient was diaphoretic, and the electrodes failed to maintain sufficient contact to produce a clear and stable tracing.

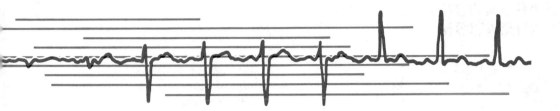

Chapter 2

ELECTROPHYSIOLOGY AND THE ELECTRICAL CONDUCTION SYSTEM

DEPOLARIZATION AND REPOLARIZATION

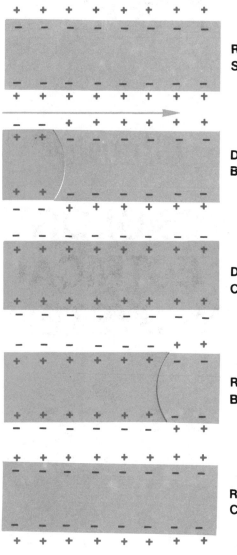

Resting State

Depolarization Beginning

Depolarization Complete

Repolarization Beginning

Repolarization Complete

The heart is composed of millions of cardiac cells, and each cell is surrounded by and filled with a solution that contains ions. As the ions move inside and across the cell membranes, a flow of electricity that produces the signals on an ECG strip is generated.

When an electrical impulse is initiated in the heart, the inside of a cardiac cell rapidly becomes positive in relation to the outside of the cell. The electrical impulse causing this excited state and this change of polarity is called *depolarization*. An electrical impulse begins at one end of a cardiac cell, and this wave of depolarization travels through the cell to the opposite end.

The return of the depolarized cardiac cell to its resting state is called *repolarization*. This phase of recovery allows the inside of the cell membrane to return to its normal negativity. Repolarization begins at the end of the cell that was just depolarized. The resting state is maintained until the arrival of the next wave of depolarization.

Once the cardiac cells have been depolarized, a second wave of depolarization cannot occur until the first depolarization is completely finished. This period is called the *absolute refractory period*. Immediately following this, the *relative refractory period* occurs during repolarization, at which time the cardiac cell is capable of being depolarized again but only by a strong stimulus.

ANATOMY

The heart is a muscular, four-chambered organ that pumps blood to all the tissues of the body and nourishes them with oxygen. The two smaller upper chambers, called the left and right atria (singular, *atrium*), are the receiving chambers and are divided by a wall called the *interatrial septum*.

The two lower chambers, called the ventricles, pump blood out of the heart and are divided by a thicker wall, called the *interventricular septum.*

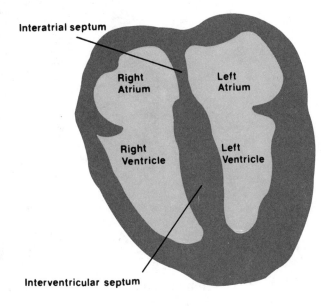

Unoxygenated blood is returned from the body to the right atrium. It flows into the right ventricle and is then pumped a short distance, via the pulmonary artery, into the lungs to become oxygenated. Once oxygenation occurs, blood enters the left atrium by way of the pulmonary veins. It flows into the left ventricle and is pumped out to the entire body via the aorta to nourish the tissues with oxygen.

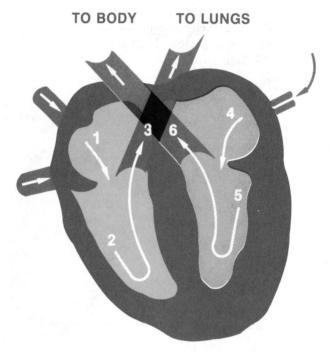

TO BODY   **TO LUNGS**

1. Unoxygenated blood returns to the right atrium from the superior and inferior venae cavae.
2. Blood proceeds to the right ventricle.
3. Blood is pumped into the pulmonary artery and into the lungs.
4. Oxygenated blood returns to the left atrium through pulmonary veins.
5. Blood flows to left ventricle.
6. Blood is pumped into the aorta and out to the body.

THE ELECTRICAL CONDUCTION SYSTEM

The electrical conduction system contains all the "wiring" and "parts" necessary to initiate and maintain rhythmic contraction of the heart. The system consists of (1) the sinoatrial (SA) node, (2) the internodal pathways, (3) the atrioventricular (AV) node, (4) the bundle of His, (5) the right bundle branch and the left bundle branch and its anterior and posterior divisions, and (7) the Purkinje fibers.

SA Node

The cardiac impulse originates in the SA node, called "the pacemaker of the heart," located in the upper wall of the right atrium.

SA NODE

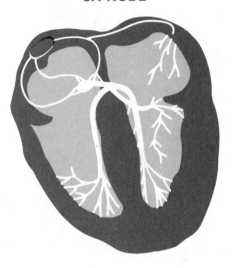

INTERNODAL PATHWAYS

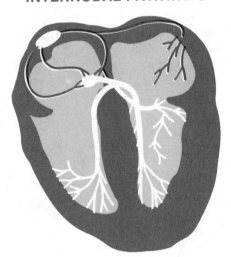

Internodal Pathways

The cardiac impulse spreads through both atria by way of the internodal pathways and causes both atria to depolarize and then to contract.

ELECTROPHYSIOLOGY AND THE ELECTRICAL CONDUCTION SYSTEM

Atrial depolarization is represented on an ECG by a *P wave*. P waves are usually upright and slightly rounded.

ATRIAL DEPOLARIZATION

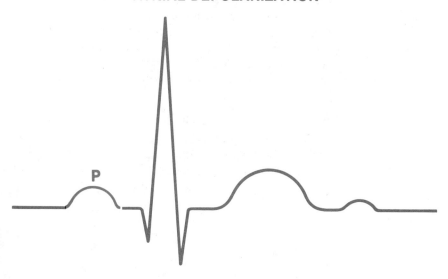

P

Remember, when cardiac cells depolarize, they must also repolarize to regain their proper resting charge. Atrial repolarization, represented by a *Ta wave*, which is in a direction opposite that of the P wave, is often not visible on an ECG because it generally coincides with another cardiac event.

AV Node

The depolarization wave arrives at the AV node, which is located on the right side of the interatrial septum; the wave is delayed at the AV node approximately .10 second before arriving at the bundle of His.

AV NODE

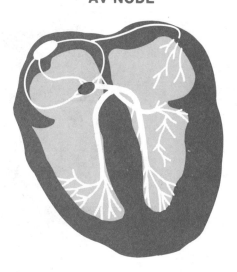

Bundle of His

The cardiac impulse spreads to the thin bundle of "threads" connecting the AV node to the bundle branches. These are located in the right side of the interatrial septum just above the ventricles.

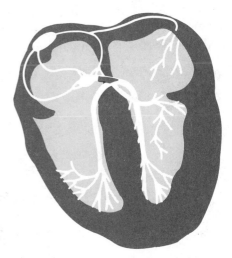

RIGHT BUNDLE BRANCH

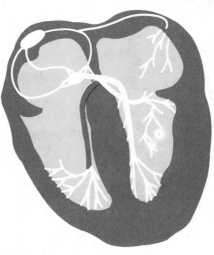

Right and Left Bundle Branches

The right bundle branch is a slender fascicle that runs along the right side of the interventricular septum and supplies the electrical impulses to the right ventricle.

The left bundle branch supplies electrical impulses to the left ventricle. It runs along the left side of the interventricular septum and divides almost immediately into an anterior and posterior division.

The Anterior Fascicle

Supplies the anterior and superior portions of the left ventricle with electrical impulses.

LEFT ANTERIOR FASCICLE

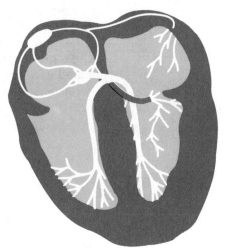

LEFT POSTERIOR FASCICLE

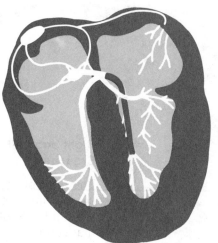

The Posterior Fascicle

Supplies the posterior and inferior portions of the left ventricle with electrical impulses.

PURKINJE FIBERS

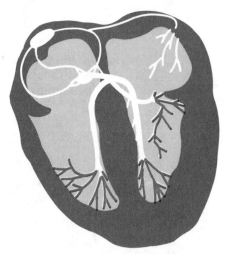

Purkinje Fibers

The bundle branches both terminate in a network of fibers located in both the left and right ventricular walls. The cardiac impulse travels into the Purkinje fibers and causes ventricular depolarization and then ventricular contraction.

Ventricular depolarization is represented by the QRS complex.

VENTRICULAR DEPOLARIZATION

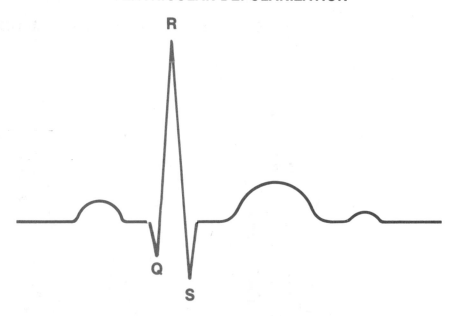

A QRS complex may be composed of a Q wave, an R wave, and an S wave, or various combinations of these waves. The point of reference on an ECG is the baseline, or isoelectric line. This is the line before the P wave. Any stylus movement above this line is positive, and any stylus movement below this line is negative.

The R wave is a positive deflection.

The Q wave is a negative deflection before an R wave.

The S wave is a negative deflection after an R wave.

R waves are always positive waves, and Q and S waves are always negative waves. We always call a ventricular depolarization complex a QRS complex whether or not all three waves are present.

It is possible to have more than one positive wave, or R wave, in a QRS complex. This second R wave is labeled R prime (R′). The repetition of an S wave is designated S prime (S′).

DIFFERENT KINDS OF QRS COMPLEXES

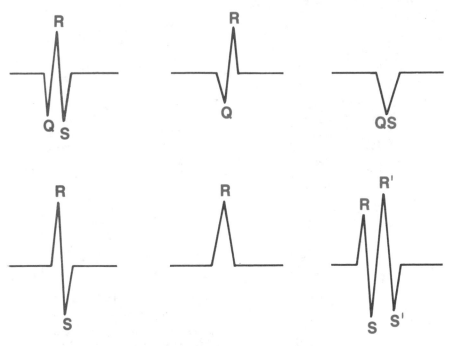

An R wave is a positive deflection.
A Q wave is a negative deflection before an R wave.
An S wave is a negative deflection after an R wave.

Ventricular repolarization is represented by the T wave. The T wave is normally upright and slightly rounded.

VENTRICULAR REPOLARIZATION

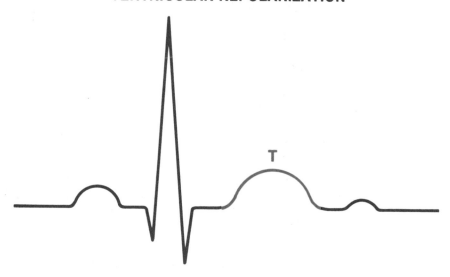

A U wave is sometimes seen after the T wave. It is thought to relate to the events of late repolarization of the ventricles. The U wave should be of the same direction as the T wave. It is important to be able to identify a U wave when it is visible so as to not confuse it with the P wave.

LATE REPOLARIZATION

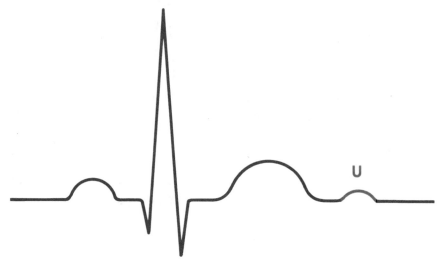

ELECTROPHYSIOLOGY AND THE ELECTRICAL CONDUCTION SYSTEM

INTERVALS AND SEGMENTS

PR Interval

The period from the beginning of the P wave to the beginning of the QRS complex is called the *PR interval*. The PR interval is routinely measured on all ECG strips.

PR Segment

The *PR segment* represents the time between the end of the P wave and the beginning of the QRS complex.

ST Segment

The distance between the end of the QRS complex (the J point) and the beginning of the T wave is called the *ST segment*. This segment is a sensitive indicator of myocardial ischemia or injury and should routinely be on the isoelectric line.

QT Interval

The time from the beginning of the QRS complex to the end of the T wave is the *QT interval*. This interval represents both ventricular depolarization and ventricular repolarization.

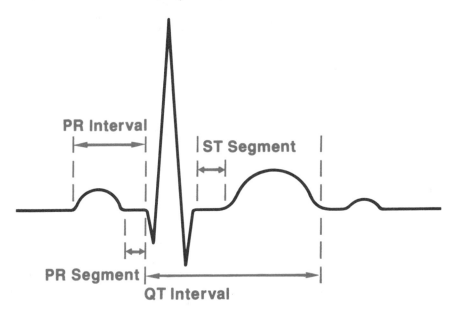

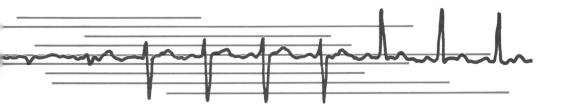

Chapter 3

ECG GRAPH PAPER AND MEASUREMENTS

TIME AND VOLTAGE

On the vertical axis of ECG graph paper we measure voltage by height in millimeters (mm). Each small square is 1 mm high, and each large square is 5 mm high.

VOLTAGE

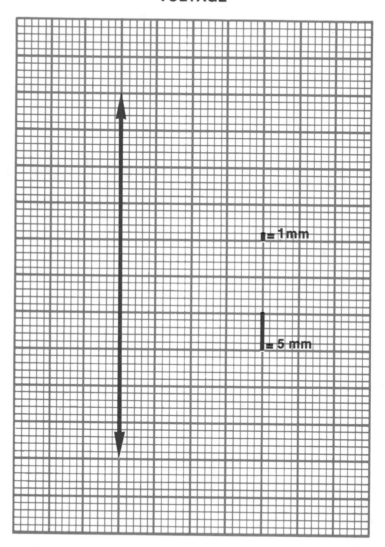

The isoelectric line is always our reference point to begin measurements. R waves are measured from the top of the isoelectric line to the top point of the R wave. Q and S waves are measured from the bottom of the isoelectric line to the bottom point of the Q or S wave.

ST elevation is measured from the top of the isoelectric line to the ST segment, and ST depression is measured from the bottom of the isoelectric line to the ST segment.

VOLTAGE MEASUREMENTS

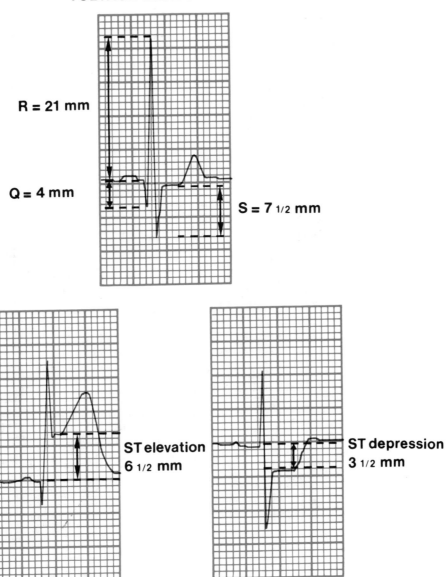

R = 21 mm

Q = 4 mm

S = 7 1/2 mm

ST elevation
6 1/2 mm

ST depression
3 1/2 mm

On the horizontal axis we measure time in seconds. Each small square is .04 second in duration, and each large square is .20 second in duration. Five large squares = 1 second (5 × .20).

TIME IN SECONDS

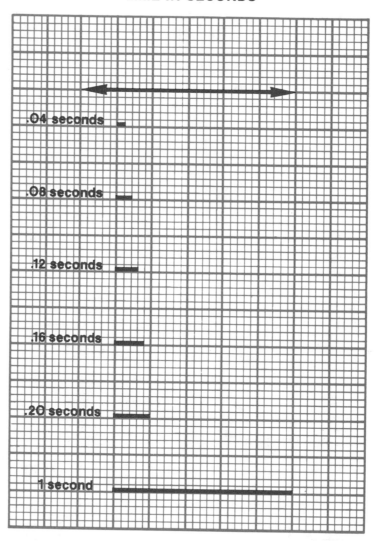

MEASUREMENTS

During our analysis of ECG strips we will be measuring PR and QRS intervals.

PR Interval

Atrial depolarization and AV conduction time are represented by the PR interval. Measurements are taken from the beginning of the P wave, where the P wave lifts off the isoelectric line, to the beginning of the first wave of the QRS complex. Count along the horizontal axis every .04 second (.04, .08, .12, .16, .20, etc.) until the correct distance between the two points is obtained; this is the PR interval in seconds. The normal range for a PR interval is .12 to .20 seconds.

PR MEASUREMENT

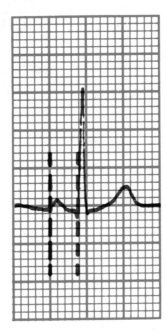

PR .14

QRS Interval

Ventricular depolarization is represented by the QRS interval. Measurements are taken from the beginning of the first wave of the QRS to the end of the last wave of the QRS. Count along the horizontal axis every .04 second until the distance between the two points is obtained; this is the QRS interval in seconds. The normal range for a QRS interval is .04 to .11 second.

QRS MEASUREMENT

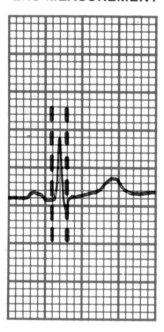

QRS .08

If you are sitting in an office and have calipers handy to make the necessary ECG measurements, life is very easy. But out in the field or in emergency situations one has to learn how to "eyeball" the measurements and make diagnoses without the luxury of time and instruments. This is easy to do with a little practice. Try to find a PR interval or QRS interval that begins on, or at least very close to, a heavy black line. (By using an interval that begins on a heavy black line, you make your point of reference easier.) Look for the end of the interval. Just eyeball how many lines to the right the interval spans and count .04, .08, and so forth until you obtain the necessary distance between the beginning and the end point of the interval.

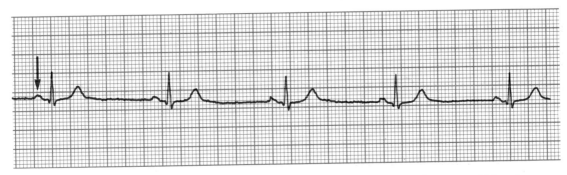

Choose the PR interval labeled with the arrow because it begins closest to a heavy black line. It extends four small boxes to the right, or .16 second.

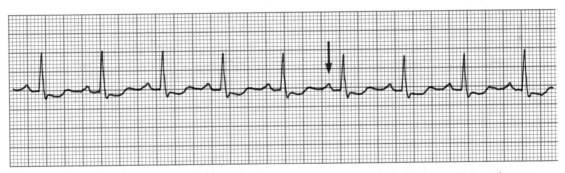

The PR interval designated with an arrow falls closest to a heavy black line. It extends five small boxes to the right, or .20 second.

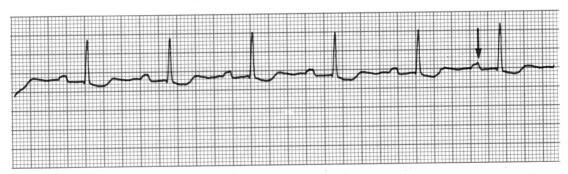

The PR interval marked with an arrow is close to a heavy black line. It extends 7½ boxes to the right, or .30 second.

ECG GRAPH PAPER AND MEASUREMENTS

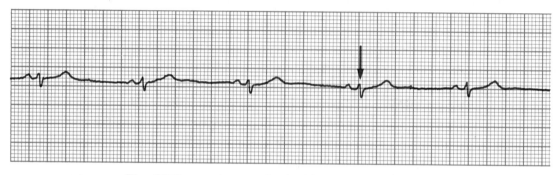

The QRS complex marked with an arrow falls closest to a heavy black line. It extends two small boxes to the right, or .08 second.

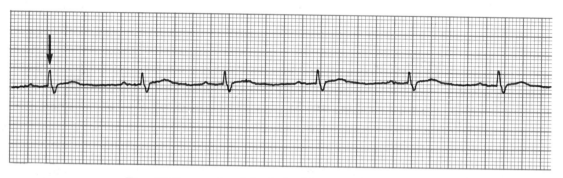

The QRS complex labeled with an arrow falls nearest to a heavy black line. It extends 2½ small boxes to the right, or .10 second.

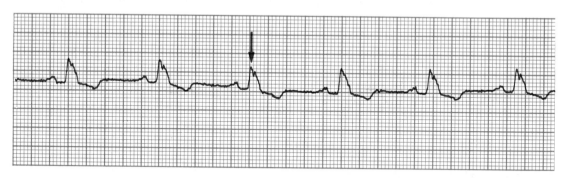

The arrow designates the QRS that falls closest to a heavy black line. The QRS extends four small boxes to the right, or .16 second.

After much practice you should be able to tell normal from abnormal measurements just by observation, even without measuring. And usually, just this distinction, rather than the exact measurement, is sufficient for monitoring.

PRACTICE ECG STRIPS

There may be a slight variation in measurements between different intervals on the same ECG strip because of patient movement or artifact. I have intentionally included artifact in some of the following ECG strips to simulate the types of recordings you might expect to find in the field. The measurements are therefore approximations. Eyeball the PR and QRS measurements rather than using calipers or rate rulers.

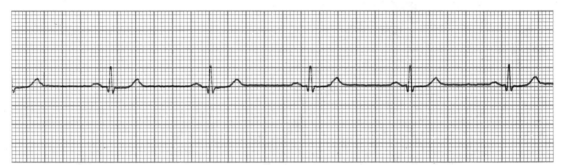

Practice strip 1

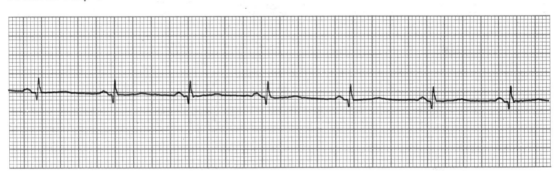

Practice strip 2

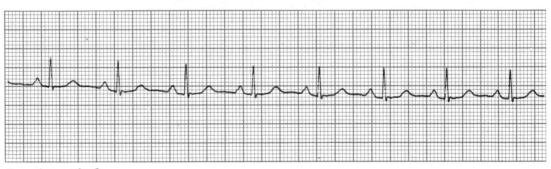

Practice strip 3

ECG GRAPH PAPER AND MEASUREMENTS

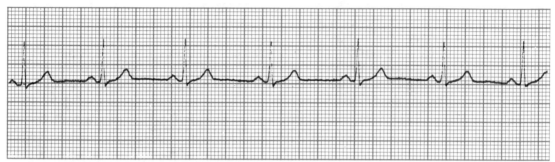

Practice strip 4

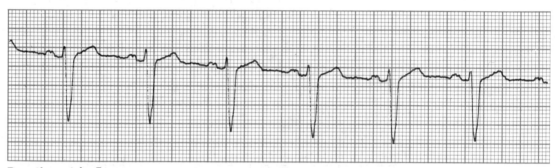

Practice strip 5

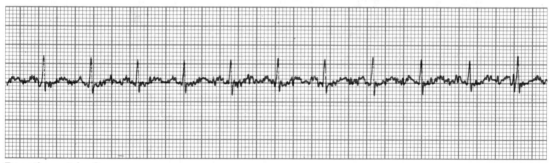

Practice strip 6

HOW TO QUICKLY AND ACCURATELY MASTER ARRHYTHMIA INTERPRETATION

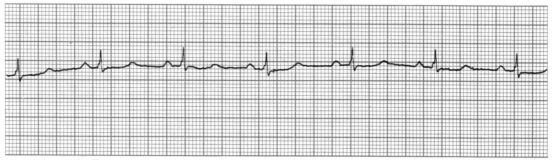

Practice strip 7

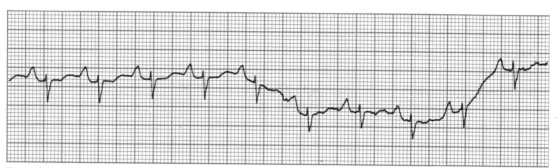

Practice strip 8

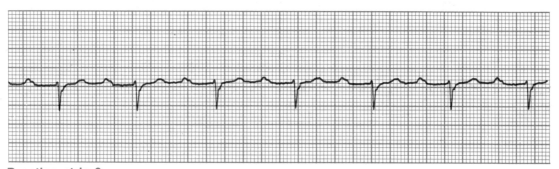

Practice strip 9

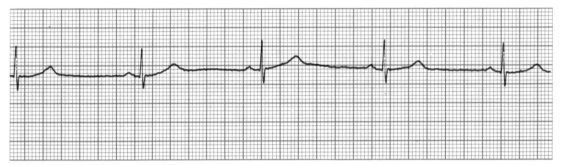

Practice strip 10

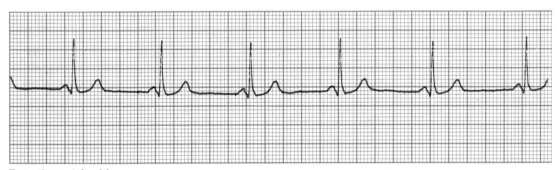

Practice strip 11

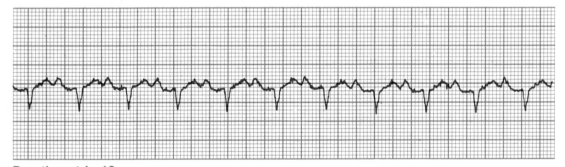

Practice strip 12

PRACTICE ECG STRIP ANSWERS

1. PR = .18   QRS = .08
2. PR = .14   QRS = .06
3. PR = .18   QRS = .06
4. PR = .16   QRS = .08
5. PR = .20   QRS = .14
6. PR = .14   QRS = .06
7. PR = .20   QRS = .08
8. PR = .20   QRS = .08
9. PR = .34   QRS = .08
10. PR = .16   QRS = .06
11. PR = .12   QRS = .08
12. PR = .24   QRS = .08

Chapter 4

DETERMINATION OF HEART RATE AND SINUS RHYTHMS

DETERMINATION OF HEART RATE

The heart rate is the number of times the heart contracts in one minute. On an ECG, the heart rate is measured from R wave to R wave (R-R cycle) to determine the ventricular rate and from P wave to P wave (P-P cycle) to determine the atrial rate. During normal sinus rhythms the atrial and ventricular rates are the same.

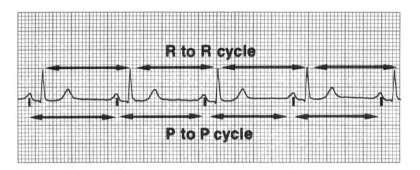

300–150–100–75–60–50–43–37–33–30

Is the easiest and quickest for rate determination. Memorize these ten numbers, and rate determination is only a step away. Choose an R wave that falls on or close to a heavy black line on the ECG paper. The first heavy black line to the right is the *300* line, the second is the *150* line, the third is the *100* line, the fourth is the *75* line, the fifth is the *60* line, the sixth is the *50* line, and so on. If the next R wave falls on the fourth heavy black line to the right, the heart rate is 75 beats per minute.

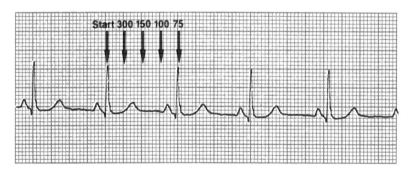

The heart rate is slightly above 75 beats per minute.

SINUS RHYTHMS

A normal heart rhythm begins in the SA node and proceeds to depolarize the atria, inscribing a P wave on the ECG. The cardiac impulse travels to the AV node and the bundle of His, then traverses the bundle branches and the Purkinje fibers; a PR interval is recorded. The impulse then reaches the ventricular muscle, and a QRS complex is displayed, representing ventricular depolarization. This is followed by an isoelectric ST segment and an upright T wave, representing ventricular repolarization. This heart rhythm is called sinus rhythm and is the normal heart rhythm. The various sinus rhythms are distinguished from one another by rate.

Sinus rhythm—60 to 100 beats per minute

Sinus bradycardia—below 60 beats per minute

Sinus tachycardia—above 100 beats per minute

Sinus arrhythmia—a slow rate (usually below 60 beats per minute), displaying an irregular R-R cycle, varying more than .16 second, and very common in children and young adults

CONDUCTION IN SINUS RHYTHM

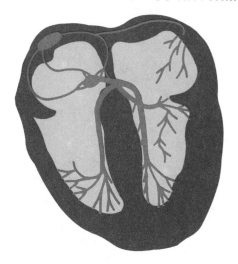

SINUS RHYTHMS

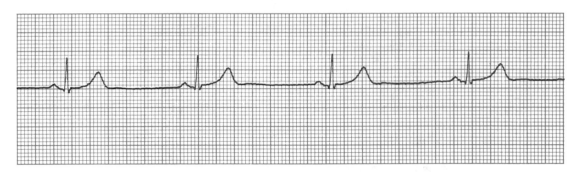

Sinus bradycardia at 43 beats per minute

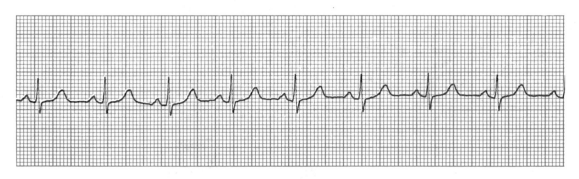

Sinus rhythm at 82 beats per minute

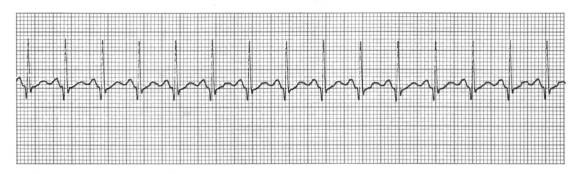

Sinus tachycardia at 149 beats per minute

SINUS ARRHYTHMIA

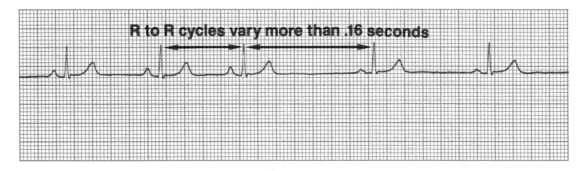

R to R cycles vary more than .16 seconds

When examining an ECG strip you should first identify the P, QRS, and T waves. Make sure you accurately identify each wave and interval on the tracing and check to see that the P-P and R-R cycles are regular. Eyeball the PR and QRS measurements, find the approximate heart rate, and identify the rhythm.

If you find that the PR measurement is less than .12 second, conduction to the ventricles may have occurred through abnormal pathways, and accelerated AV conduction is present. If the PR measurement is greater than .20 second, there is a delay in conduction through the AV node and first degree AV block is present. Neither of these abnormalities is particularly significant during routine monitoring.

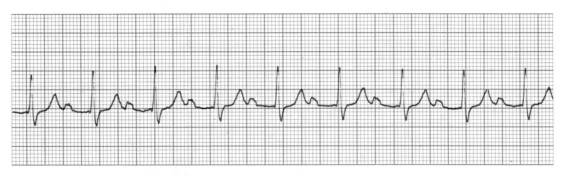

Sinus rhythm with first degree AV block. The PR interval is longer than .20 second.

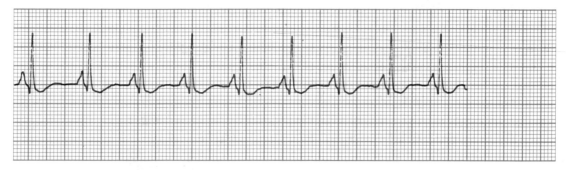

Sinus tachycardia with accelerated AV conduction. The PR interval is less than .12 second.

If you find your measurements for the QRS complex to be greater than the normal range of .11 second, a *bundle branch block* is present. One of the bundle branches can no longer carry electrical impulses to its respective ventricle. The impulses from the functioning bundle branch must depolarize its own ventricle first, and then send electrical impulses to the electrically inoperative ventricle. Because of the abnormal path of conduction and the resultant delay, a widened QRS is recorded. When one-lead monitoring is used, it is difficult to distinguish which bundle branch is not functioning, so the general term *bundle branch block* is used to cover either abnormality.

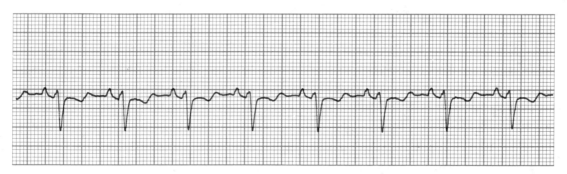

The P-P and R-R cycles are regular, and the PR interval is constant. The QRS complexes are greater than .11 second, confirming the diagnosis of sinus rhythm with a bundle branch block.

Bundle branch block may be permanent, may occur transiently, or may be rate related. As the heart rate increases, one of the bundle branches becomes unable to repolarize as rapidly as necessary, and a rate-related bundle branch block occurs. Intermittently, as the heart rate increases, the QRS complex widens to greater than .11 second and then returns to its normal duration as the heart rate slows.

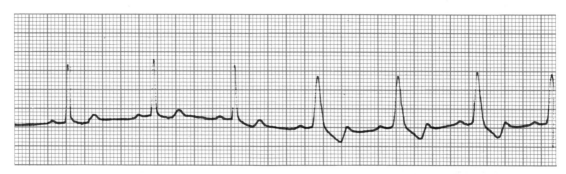

Sinus rhythm with intermittent, rate-related bundle branch block. The PR interval and the P-P and R-R cycles remain constant. The only change is the widening of the QRS complex midway through the strip, demonstrating an intermittent bundle branch block.

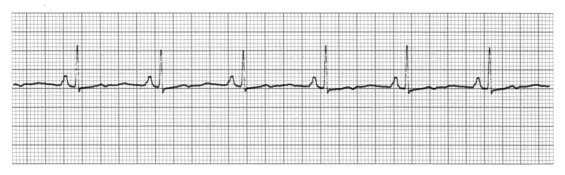

The P-P and R-R cycles are regular. The PR is .14 second, the QRS is .06 second, and the heart rate is 65 beats per minute, demonstrating sinus rhythm.

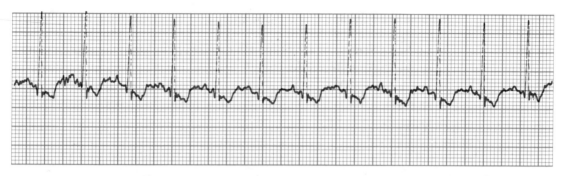

The P-P and R-R cycles are regular. The PR is .14 second, and the QRS is .08 second. Because of the rate of 120 beats per minute, sinus tachycardia is diagnosed.

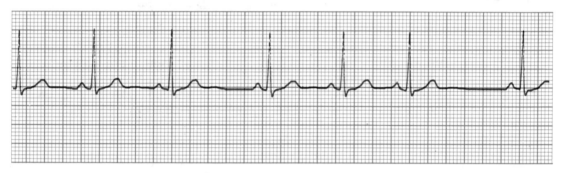

The P-P and R-R cycles vary, but each is preceded by a constant PR of .16 second and a QRS of .08 second. Sinus arrhythmia is diagnosed because of the variation in the P-P and R-R cycles.

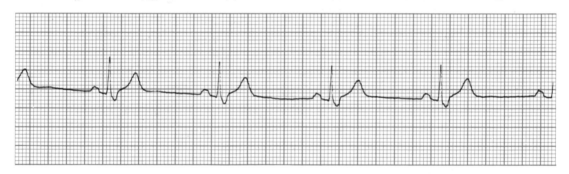

The P-P and R-R cycles are regular, and each QRS of .12 second is preceded by a constant PR of .18 second. Sinus bradycardia with a bundle branch block is present at 50 beats per minute.

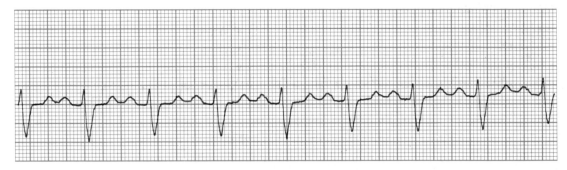

The P-P and R-R cycles are regular, the PR is .24 second, and the QRS is .14 second. The heart rate is 85 beats per minute, demonstrating sinus rhythm with first degree AV block and bundle branch block.

Identification of complexes and intervals is made more difficult when artifact is present. If a P wave or QRS or PR interval cannot be identified or measured in one complex, the entire tracing should be scanned to find suitable intervals. If a tracing is absolutely unreadable, a guesswork interpretation should not be attempted.

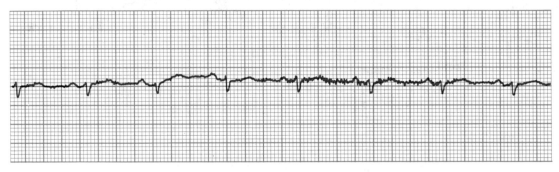

The complexes are small, and some are distorted by artifact, but measurements are still possible. The PR is .18 second, the QRS is .06 second, and the P-P and R-R cycles appear regular. The rhythm is sinus at approximately 80 beats per minute.

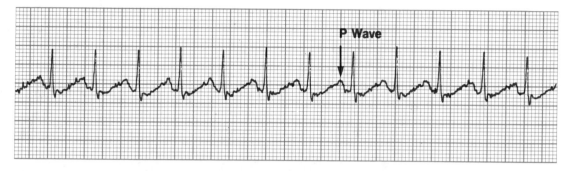

The rapid rate and the slight baseline artifact make interpretation slightly difficult. Make certain that you accurately identify all the waves and intervals before you begin measurements. The P wave is visible on the descending limb of the T wave. The PR is .14 second, and the QRS is .08 second. Sinus tachycardia is present at approximately 130 beats per minute.

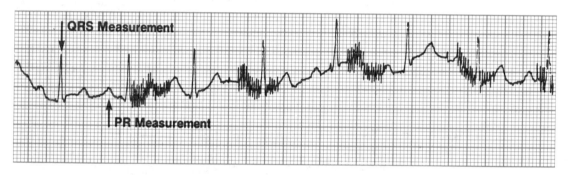

Although the artifact distorts much of the tracing, P waves and QRS complexes are still visible. The PR is .24 second, the QRS is .08 second, and the P-P and R-R cycles appear fairly regular at 75 beats per minute. This strip represents sinus rhythm with first degree AV block.

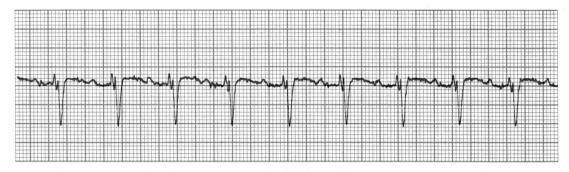

Although much baseline artifact distorts this strip, measurements are possible. The PR is .26, the QRS is .14, and the P-P and R-R cycles appear regular. This strip represents sinus rhythm at 100 beats per minute with first degree AV block and a bundle branch block.

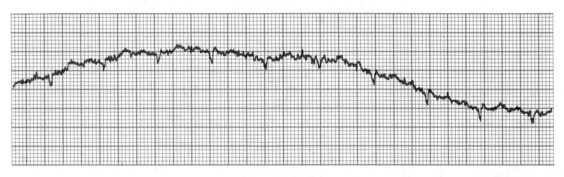

Artifact makes identification of P waves impossible. The QRS is approximately .08 second. The R-R cycle is regular at 100 beats per minute, but without P wave identification accurate rhythm analysis is impossible.

PRACTICE ECG STRIPS

There may be a slight variation in measurements between different intervals on the same ECG strip due to patient movement or artifact. I have purposely included artifact in some of the ECG strips to simulate the types of strips you might expect to find in the field, and the measurements will therefore be approximations. Eyeball the PR, QRS, and heart rate, and identify the heart rhythm.

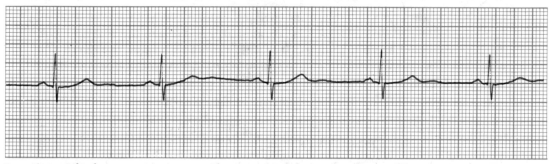

Practice strip 1

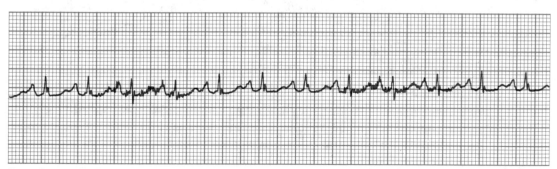

Practice strip 2

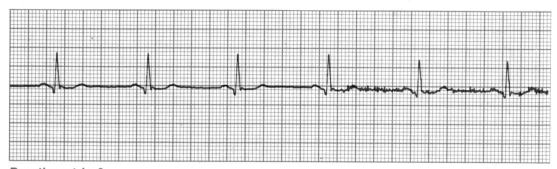

Practice strip 3

HOW TO QUICKLY AND ACCURATELY MASTER ARRHYTHMIA INTERPRETATION

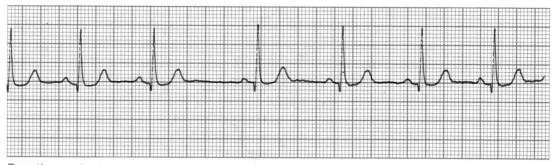

Practice strip 4

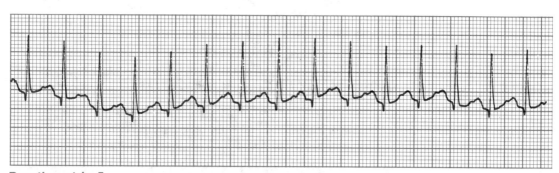

Practice strip 5

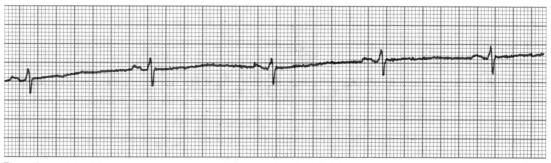

Practice strip 6

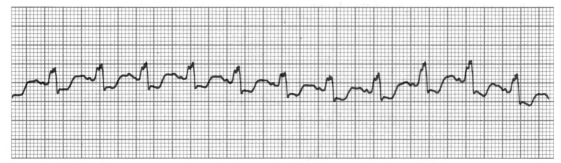

Practice strip 7

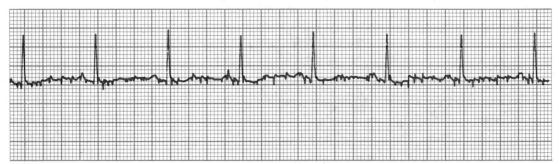

Practice strip 8

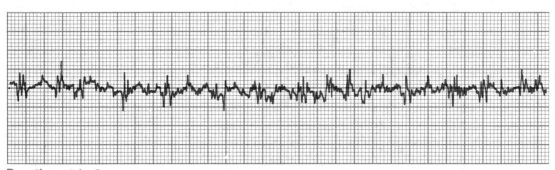

Practice strip 9

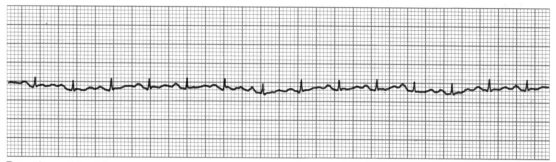

Practice strip 10

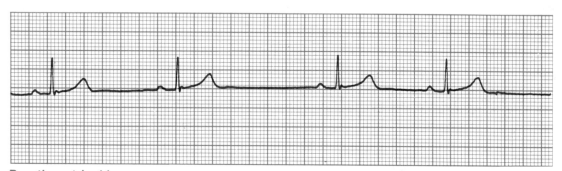

Practice strip 11

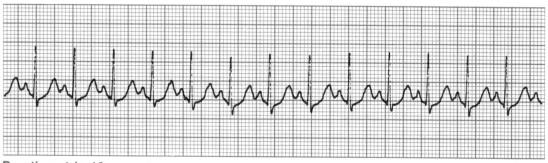

Practice strip 12

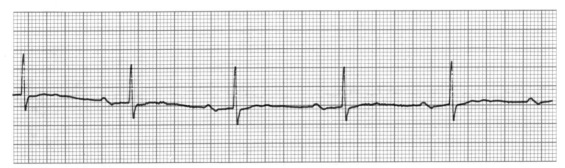

Practice strip 13

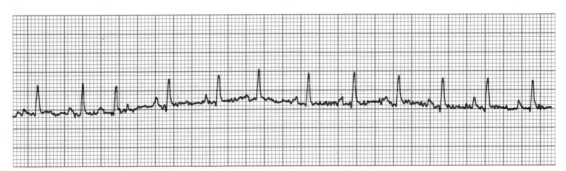

Practice strip 14

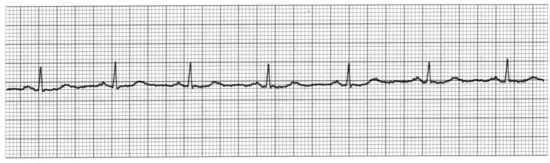

Practice strip 15

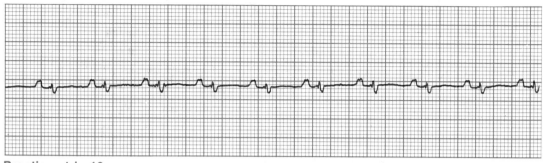

Practice strip 16

PRACTICE ECG STRIP ANSWERS

1. PR = .16   QRS = .06   Rate = 50   Rhythm = sinus bradycardia

2. PR = .16   QRS = .06   Rate = 135   Rhythm = sinus tachycardia

3. PR = .14   QRS = .08   Rate = 60   Rhythm = sinus rhythm

4. PR = .16   QRS = .10   Rate = Varies   Rhythm = sinus arrhythmia

5. PR = .16   QRS = .08   Rate = 150   Rhythm = sinus tachycardia

6. PR = .16   QRS = .08   Rate = 50   Rhythm = sinus bradycardia

7. PR = .14   QRS = .12   Rate = 125   Rhythm = sinus tachycardia with bundle branch block

8. PR = .16   QRS = .06   Rate = 75   Rhythm = sinus rhythm

9. PR = ?   QRS = ?   Rate = ?   Rhythm = ?

10. PR = .12   QRS = .05   Rate = 150   Rhythm = sinus tachycardia

11. PR = .20   QRS = .06   Rate = 43   Rhythm = sinus arrhythmia

12. PR = .12   QRS = .06   Rate = 140   Rhythm = sinus tachycardia

13. PR = .30   QRS = .08   Rate = 53   Rhythm = sinus bradycardia with first degree AV block

14. PR = .14   QRS = .08   Rate = 125   Rhythm = sinus tachycardia

15. PR = .18   QRS = .06   Rate = 70   Rhythm = sinus rhythm

16. PR = .16   QRS = .08   Rate = 100   Rhythm = sinus rhythm

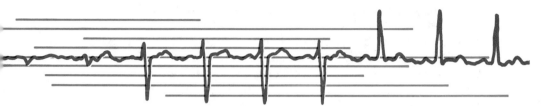

Chapter 5

PREMATURE
CONTRACTIONS

The sinus node is the pacemaker of the heart and usually regulates the heart's rhythm. But other areas in the atria, AV node, and ventricles are also capable of pacemaker activity and can cause extra heartbeats to occur during the heart's normal rhythm. These extra beats, called premature contractions, extrasystoles, or ectopic beats, are named according to the area where they originate—atrial, AV nodal, or ventricular. Those that originate either in the atria or in the AV node are called *supraventricular* beats—meaning "above the ventricles"—and those that originate from the ventricles are called ventricular.

ATRIAL PREMATURE CONTRACTION

An atrial premature contraction (APC) originates anywhere in the atria other than the SA node, and it occurs earlier than expected during the normal P-P cycle. Once the APC depolarizes the atria, in a direction slightly different from normal, thereby causing a different-looking P wave, it follows the normal conduction pathways through the remainder of the heart, recording a QRS complex identical to the sinus QRS complex. An APC is followed by a pause as the sinus node takes time to recover from the electrical impulses of the APC and to reset its cycle to resume its regular pacemaking rhythm.

APCs can occur as isolated beats, or they can occur as pairs or in runs of APCs. Six or more APCs in a row constitute an atrial rhythm (discussed in Chapter 7).

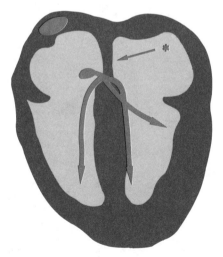

The following simplified criteria are used for recognition of an APC:

1. An APC is early.
2. The ectopic P wave (one arising from an abnormal site) looks different from sinus P wave.
3. The ectopic QRS usually resembles the QRS of a normal cardiac rhythm.

When beginning to interpret an ECG strip, you must first accurately identify all the waves, complexes, and intervals and check the P-P and R-R cycles for regularity. Only in this way can you immediately identify a premature beat followed by its expected pause. Take eyeball measurements of the PR and QRS intervals to ascertain that they are within normal limits. Then find the heart rate and identify the heart rhythm. Be sure to take the measurements from the basic cardiac rhythm and not the premature beats.

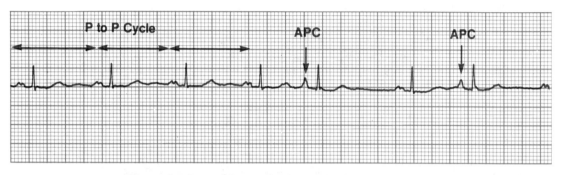

Sinus rhythm with two isolated APCs. The APCs arrive early in relation to the normal P-P cycle. Note the difference in configuration of the ectopic P waves compared with the sinus P waves. Each APC is followed by a pause as the sinus node resets itself to begin its rhythm once again.

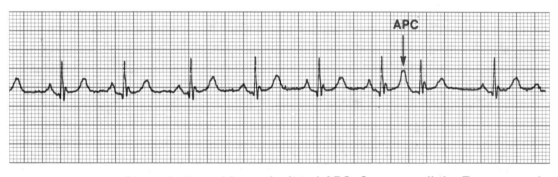

Sinus rhythm with one isolated APC. Compare all the T waves and notice how the early ectopic P wave of the APC distorts the T wave of the previous beat. On scanning the strip, note the regularity of the P-P and R-R cycles until the APC arrives. You should learn to immediately pick out the beat or beats that are out of step with the remainder of the strip.

PREMATURE CONTRACTIONS

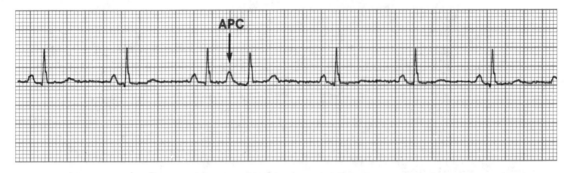

Sinus rhythm with one isolated APC. Because of the slow sinus rate it is easy to spot the early beat and the pause following it. Train your eyes to pick out any irregularity or pattern in the rhythm.

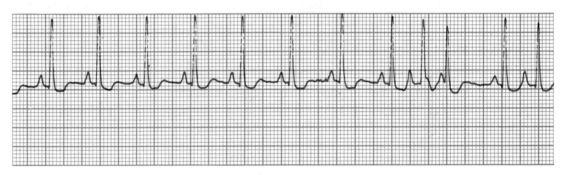

Sinus tachycardia with a pair of APCs and an isolated APC

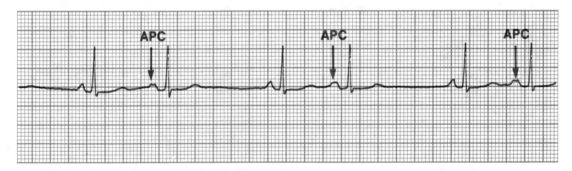

Sinus bradycardia with APCs occuring every other beat (bigeminy). Notice how alternate beats are early and have P waves different in configuration from those of the sinus P waves. You should recognize the pattern of bigeminy immediately when scanning this strip.

HOW TO QUICKLY AND ACCURATELY MASTER ARRHYTHMIA INTERPRETATION

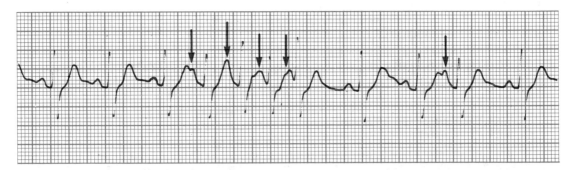

Sinus tachycardia with four APCs in a row and an isolated APC. The ectopic P waves distort the T waves of the previous beats and are labeled with arrows to help in identification. First, scan the P-P and R-R cycles, noting the irregularity, and begin to identify the sinus cycle by finding the beats with the constant PR interval and the P waves with the identical configurations. Estimate the PR, QRS, and rate and label the heart rhythm. Then begin to identify the arrhythmias. There are short R-R cycles followed by long R-R cycles, which characterize the premature arrival of APCs followed by pauses to enable the sinus node to recover from the premature beat.

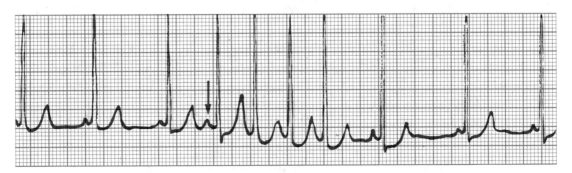

Sinus rhythm with a run of five APCs in a row and then returning to sinus rhythm. The first APC in the run is indicated by an arrow.

If an APC comes so early in the cardiac cycle that the ectopic P wave falls on the early part of the T wave of the previous beat, the impulse may find the AV node still busy or refractory from the previous beat and be unable to conduct the ectopic P wave to the ventricles to produce a QRS complex. Only an early ectopic P wave is recorded, followed by a pause. This is termed a *nonconducted APC*.

PREMATURE CONTRACTIONS

The following simplified criterion is used for recognition of a nonconducted APC:

1. An early ectopic P wave with no QRS complex, followed by a pause.

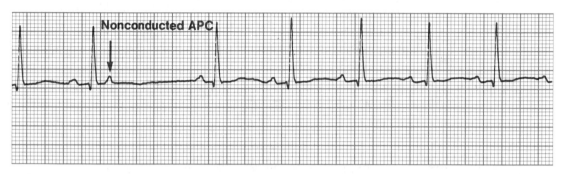

Sinus rhythm with first degree AV block and one nonconducted APC. The ectopic P wave distorts the T wave of the preceding beat and is followed by a pause while the sinus node resets. The APC arrived too early to be conducted through the AV node to the ventricles to produce a QRS complex.

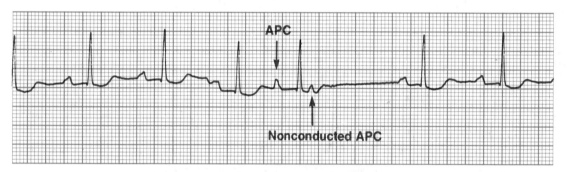

Sinus rhythm with first degree AV block and one isolated APC followed immediately by a nonconducted APC. The second ectopic P wave came too early in the cycle to be conducted through the AV node to the ventricles because the AV node was still refractory from the previous beat.

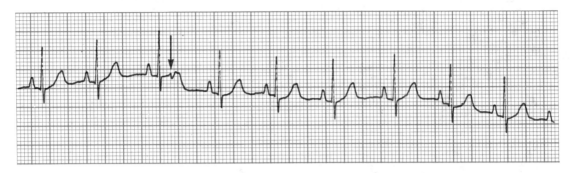

Is the arrow pointing to a nonconducted APC hidden in the T wave? If this were a nonconducted APC, it would be followed by a significant pause as the sinus node recovers from a premature depolarization and resets its cycle. There is no pause, and the R-R cycle continues on regularly. This represents artifact on the ECG rather than an arrhythmia.

AV NODAL OR JUNCTIONAL PREMATURE CONTRACTION

A junctional (or nodal) premature contraction (JPC or NPC) arises from the tissue in or surrounding the AV node and occurs as an early beat preceded by an inverted P wave, followed by an inverted P wave, or demonstrating no visible P wave because it is buried within the QRS complex. The inverted P wave represents atrial depolarization from a reverse direction (retrograde, from the AV node back up to the atria rather than from the sinus node down toward the AV node). Because further conduction to the ventricles proceeds through normal conduction pathways, the QRS usually resembles that of the normal cardiac rhythm. The JPC is followed by a pause as the sinus node takes time to recover from the electrical impulses of the JPC and to reset its cycle to begin its regular pacemaking rhythm again.

JPCs can occur as isolated beats, or they can occur as pairs or in runs of JPCs. Six or more JPCs in a row constitute a junctional rhythm (discussed in Chapter 7)

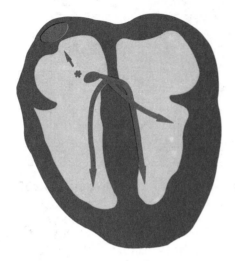

The following simplified criteria are used for recognition of a JPC:

1. The JPC is early.
2. The ectopic P wave is inverted either before or after the QRS complex or is not visible at all.
3. The QRS usually resembles the QRS of a normal cardiac rhythm.

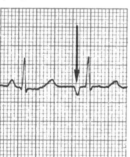

JPC with inverted P wave preceding QRS

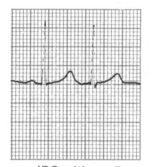

JPC with no P wave visible

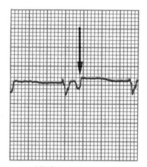

JPC with inverted P wave following QRS

As with APCs, JPCs may also be nonconducted. An early inverted P wave without a QRS complex following it is recorded on or immediately after a T wave and is followed by a ventricular pause.

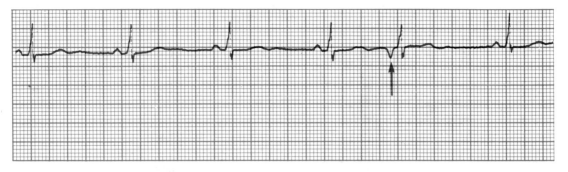

Sinus bradycardia with one isolated JPC. Note the inverted P wave preceding the QRS.

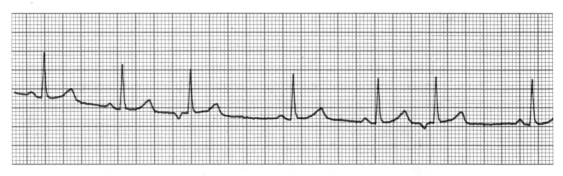

Sinus rhythm with JPCs every third beat (trigeminy)

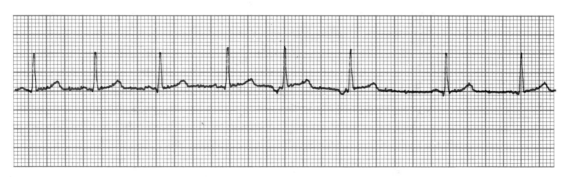

Sinus rhythm with a pair of JPCs

PREMATURE CONTRACTIONS

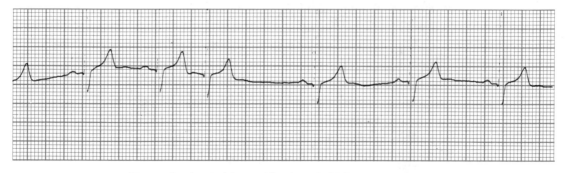

Sinus rhythm with one isolated JPC and no visible inverted ectopic P waves either preceding or following the QRS complex

VENTRICULAR PREMATURE CONTRACTION

A ventricular premature contraction (VPC) is an early beat that arises from an area of the ventricles. It depolarizes the ventricle where it originates and then proceeds to depolarize the other ventricle. Because conduction through the ventricles is not occurring through the designated conduction pathways, but rather through ventricular muscle, the conduction is slower than normal and produces a widened and different-looking QRS complex. The ventricles depolarize first, inscribing a widened QRS, while the atrial cycle usually continues independently, uninterrupted by the VPC.

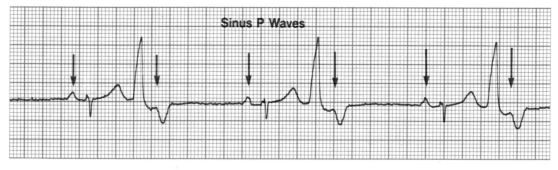

Sinus rhythm with VPCs in bigeminy. Notice how the sinus P-P cycle continues at a regular rate undisturbed by the VPCs.

If the VPCs all originate from the same area, or focus, in the ventricles, they are called *unifocal VPCs* and have the same configuration. If the VPCs arise from multiple foci in the ventricles, they are called *multifocal VPCs* and vary in their configurations.

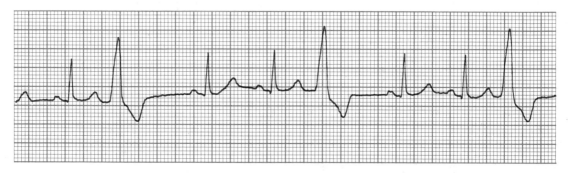

Sinus rhythm with three unifocal VPCs in trigeminy

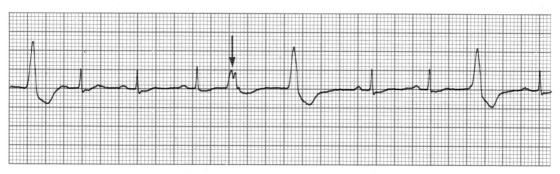

Sinus rhythm with multifocal VPCs—two isolated and one pair. The VPC identified by the arrow is from a different focus.

End Diastolic VPC

A VPC that occurs immediately after the atria have depolarized from a sinus impulse but before conduction to the ventricles occurs is an *end diastolic VPC*. A sinus P wave is either partially or completely inscribed, followed immediately by a VPC. The sinus P wave has no relationship to the VPC. Each has occurred independently and almost concurrently.

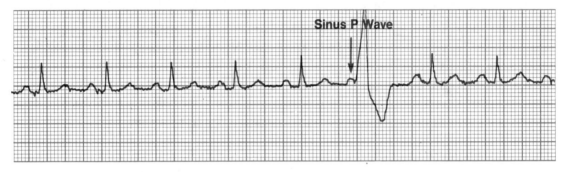

Sinus rhythm with one end diastolic VPC. The VPC immediately follows the sinus P wave but bears no relationship to it.

If the end diastolic VPC occurs slightly later in the cycle after the sinus P wave has been fully inscribed on the ECG, then a *fusion beat* may occur and would be a combination of both an end diastolic VPC and a sinus beat. The electrical activity in both the sinus node and the ventricles has occurred almost concurrently, and the fusion beat is a product of electrical impulses from both chambers. It has no more significance than an end diastolic VPC. Its QRS will resemble both the VPC and the QRS complex of the sinus rhythm.

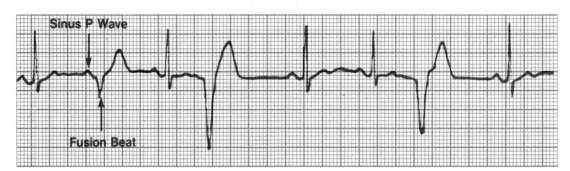

Sinus rhythm with two isolated unifocal VPCs and one fusion beat. The sinus P wave is fully inscribed. This permits the following QRS to be composed of electrical impulses from both the sinus node and the ventricle.

Interpolated VPC

A VPC that is sandwiched between two sinus beats with no pause following it is an *interpolated VPC*.

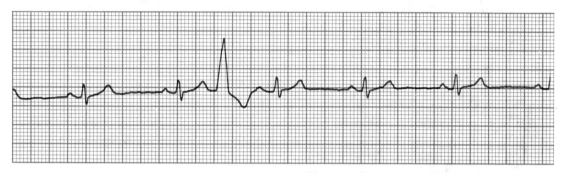

Sinus rhythm with one interpolated VPC. The VPC is sandwiched between two sinus beats with no pause following it. The P-P and R-R cycles remain fairly regular.

Malignant VPC

A VPC that falls on the T wave of the previous beat and makes the heart vulnerable to repetitive firing of the ventricular focus is called a *malignant VPC*.

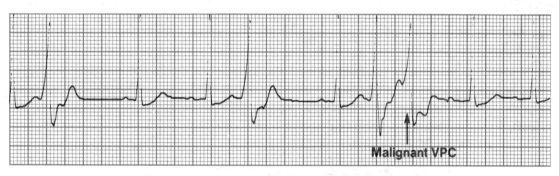

Sinus rhythm with four unifocal VPCs—two isolated and one pair. The second VPC in the pair is malignant because it falls on the T wave of the previous VPC.

VPCs can occur as isolated beats, or they can occur as pairs or in runs of VPCs. Six or more VPCs in a row constitute a ventricular rhythm (discussed in Chapter 8).

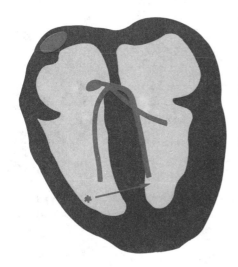

The following simplified criteria are used for recognition of a VPC:

1. The VPC is early.
2. The QRS is wide (.12 second or greater) and looks different from the QRS of the normal cardiac rhythm.
3. No ectopic P wave is present. Although the sinus P wave may occur directly before or after the VPC, it bears no relationship to it.

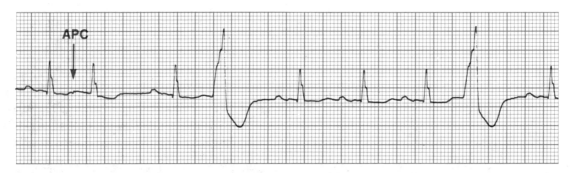

Sinus rhythm with first degree AV block and one isolated APC and two isolated unifocal VPCs. The VPCs are easy to identify, but the APC could be missed. Scan the strip for an initial impression. Identify the P waves, PR intervals, and QRS complexes, eyeball the PR and QRS measurements, check for regularity of the P-P and R-R cycles, and identify the rate and rhythm. Start at the left side of the strip and move rightward, labeling each beat and pause that occurs until you are certain that the interpretation you have chosen meets all the criteria.

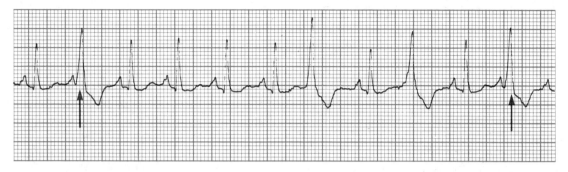

Sinus tachycardia with four isolated unifocal VPCs. Two are end diastolic (*arrows*). Notice the sinus P wave preceding each.

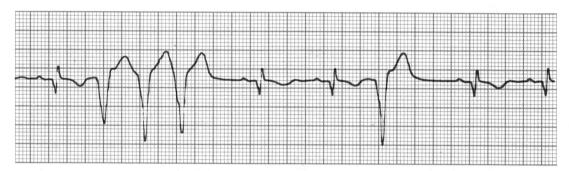

Sinus rhythm with four unifocal VPCs—one isolated and three in a row. The third VPC is malignant.

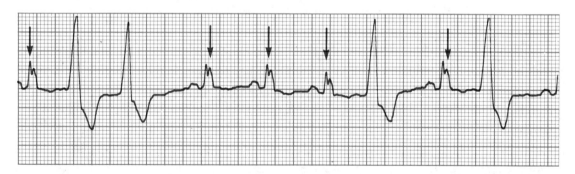

Sinus rhythm with bundle branch block and four unifocal VPCs—two isolated and one pair. Be careful that you accurately identify the widened QRS complexes of bundle branch block (*arrows*). Notice how they are all preceded by a sinus P wave with a constant PR interval. Always identify the basic rhythm first and eyeball the measurements. Then begin to label any abnormalities.

PREMATURE CONTRACTIONS

DIFFERENTIAL DIAGNOSIS

APCs or sinus arrhythmia?

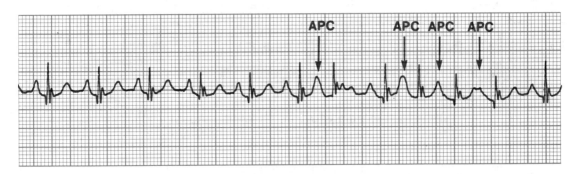

In a strip with a rapid rate such as this, it is often difficult to get your bearings. Because of the irregular P-P and R-R cycle an initial impression would be either APCs or sinus arrhythmia. The PR and QRS measurements are normal, and the first few beats can be distinguished as sinus tachycardia because of the regularity of rhythm and the constant PR interval. An early beat occurs, with its ectopic P wave distorting the previous T wave. This beat is followed by a pause and then a sinus beat. Three early beats occur in a row, each preceded by ectopic P waves with configurations different from that of the sinus P wave. This confirms the diagnosis of APCs and rules out sinus arrhythmia.

Sinus arrhythmia or nonconducted APC?

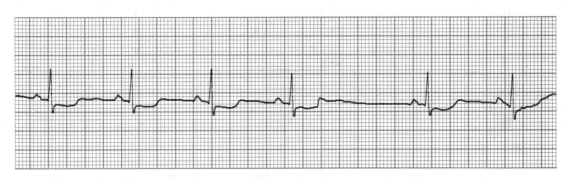

Check the T wave preceding the pause and note the appearance of an ectopic P wave. This confirms the diagnosis of sinus rhythm with one nonconducted APC and rules out sinus arrhythmia.

Sinus arrhythmia or nonconducted APC?

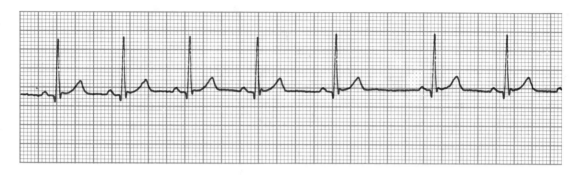

The T wave preceding the pause shows no evidence of the ectopic
P wave of an APC. This rules out a nonconducted APC and
demonstrates the waxing and waning of the heart rhythm during
sinus arrhythmia.

Sinus tachycardia with nonconducted APCs in trigeminy or sinus
bradycardia with APCs in bigeminy?

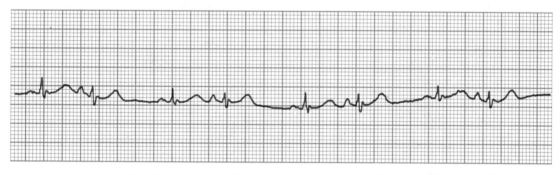

The first beat of the strip begins with a flattened P wave. The
second beat displays an upright P wave unlike that of the sinus
beat, so we can rule out two sinus beats in a row or sinus
tachycardia. This ectopic beat is followed by a pause, and then the
cycle repeats itself. This strip represents sinus rhythm with APCs in
bigeminy.

PREMATURE CONTRACTIONS

End diastolic VPC or intermittent bundle branch block?

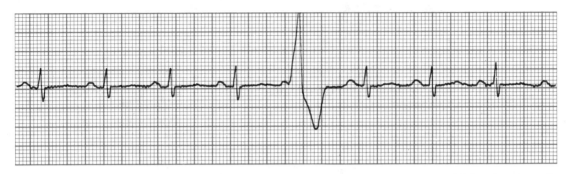

Sinus rhythm is present with one wide and bizarre QRS. This beat is preceded by a sinus P wave, but the PR interval is visibly shorter than the sinus beats, confirming the diagnosis of end diastolic VPC. If this were intermittent bundle branch block, the PR interval of the widened QRS would be the same as those of the sinus beats.

PRACTICE ECG STRIPS

I have purposely included artifact in some of the ECG strips to simulate the types of strips you might expect to find in the field. Eyeball the PR and QRS intervals for normal or abnormal intervals rather than exact measurements, estimate the rate, identify the rhythm, and label any arrhythmias present.

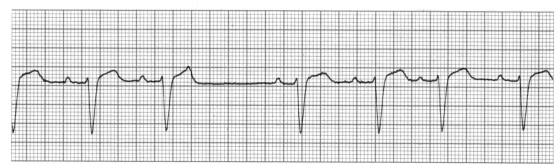

Practice strip 1

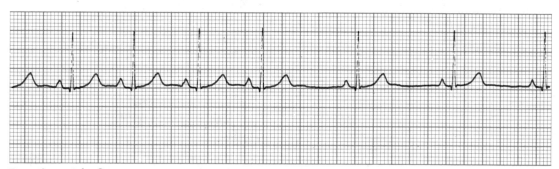

Practice strip 2

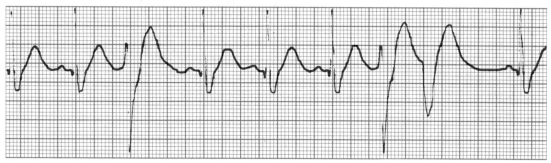

Practice strip 3

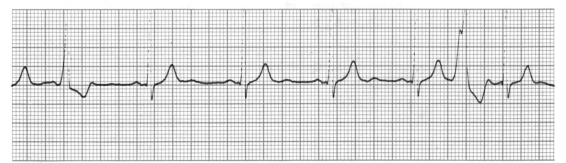

Practice strip 4

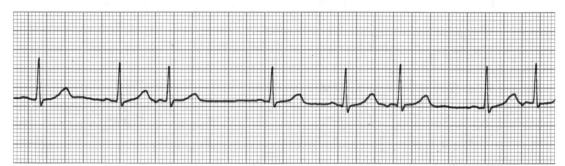

Practice strip 5

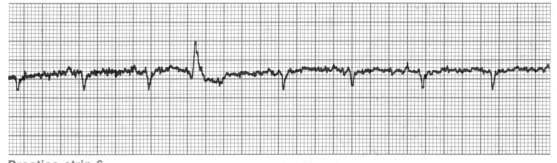

Practice strip 6

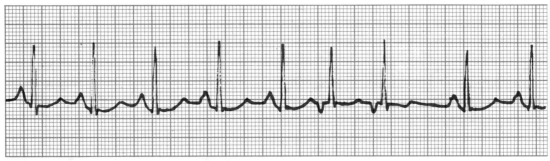

Practice strip 7

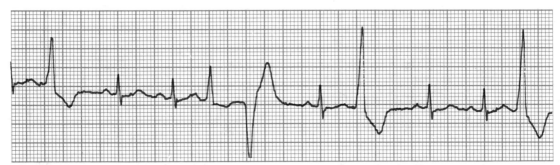

Practice strip 8

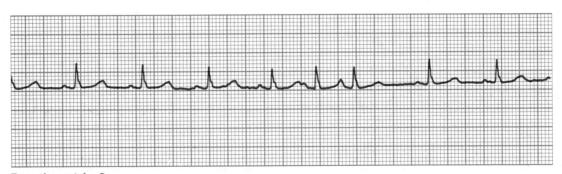

Practice strip 9

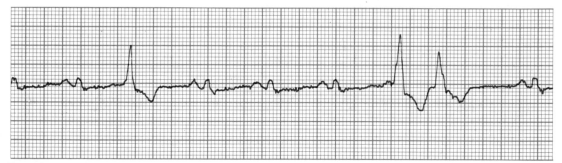

Practice strip 10

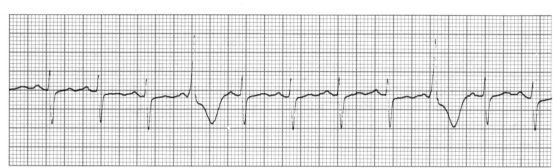

Practice strip 11

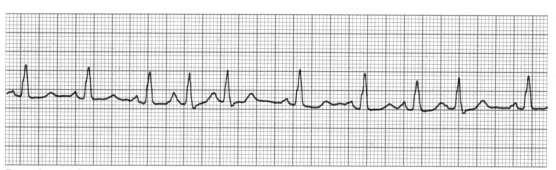

Practice strip 12

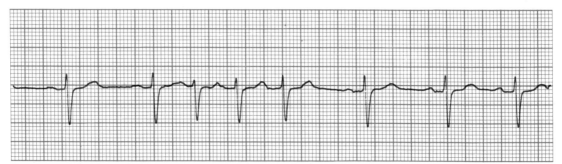

Practice strip 13

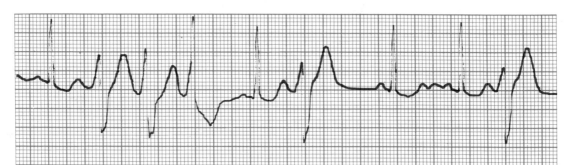

Practice strip 14

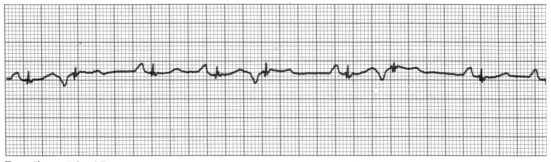

Practice strip 15

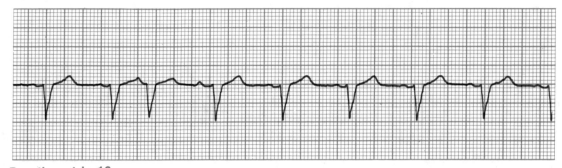

Practice strip 16

PRACTICE ECG STRIP ANSWERS

1. Sinus rhythm with first degree AV block and bundle branch block with one nonconducted APC and one isolated APC

2. Sinus arrhythmia

3. Sinus rhythm with bundle branch block and multifocal VPCs— one isolated and one pair

4. Sinus rhythm with two isolated unifocal VPCs–the first one a fusion beat and the second one interpolated

5. Sinus rhythm with three isolated JPCs

6. Probable sinus rhythm with one isolated VPC

7. Sinus rhythm with a pair of JPCs

8. Sinus rhythm with five multifocal VPCs—three isolated and one pair

9. Sinus rhythm with a pair of APCs

10. Sinus rhythm with bundle branch block and three unifocal VPCs—one isolated and one pair. The first VPC in the pair is end diastolic.

11. Sinus tachycardia with two isolated unifocal end diastolic VPCs

12. Sinus rhythm with two pairs of APCs

13. Sinus rhythm with three APCs in a row

14. Sinus rhythm with multifocal VPCs—three in a row and two isolated VPCs

15. Sinus rhythm with three isolated JPCs

16. Sinus rhythm with one isolated APC

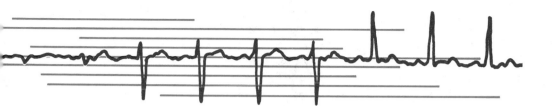

Chapter 6

ESCAPE BEATS
AND RHYTHMS

An escape beat is always late in relation to the normal R-R cycle. When the pacemaker of the heart does not fire, the escape mechanism rescues the heart from uncomfortable or dangerous ventricular pauses. An escape beat may occur after the pause following a premature contraction or after longer pauses caused by more serious arrhythmias discussed in later chapters. It is important to discover what arrhythmia has caused the pause and escape beat.

Escape beats may be isolated or may occur up to five in a row. Six or more escape beats in a row constitute an escape rhythm, discussed later in this chapter.

JUNCTIONAL ESCAPE BEAT

The most common type of escape beat arises from the AV node. When a pause occurs in the heart, the AV node issues a response, and a junctional escape beat is recorded. The impulse travels from the AV node down normal conduction pathways and records a QRS complex like that of the normal cardiac rhythm. The electrical impulse also travels retrogradely to depolarize the atria and inscribes an inverted P wave immediately before, after, or in the middle of the junctional escape beat. Often the sinus node resumes pacemaker activity again after the pause and is interrupted by a junctional escape beat before conduction to the ventricles occurs. This is seen as a sinus P wave with a shortened PR interval.

Junctional escape beats can occur as isolated beats, or they can occur as pairs or in runs.

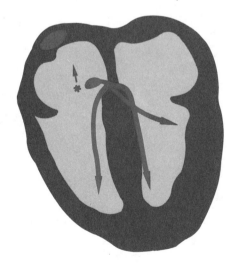

The following simplified criteria are used for recognition of a junctional escape beat:

1. A junctional escape beat is late in relation to the normal R-R cycle.
2. It is preceded by an inverted P wave, no P wave, or a sinus P wave with shortened PR interval.
3. The QRS usually resembles the QRS of a normal cardiac rhythm.

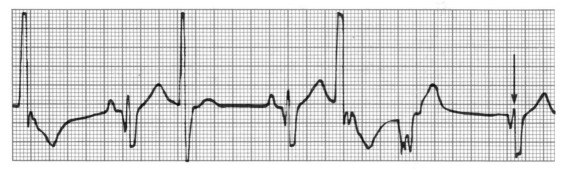

Sinus rhythm with bundle branch block and four multifocal VPCs in bigeminy. Three are isolated, and there is one pair. The pair is followed by a junctional escape beat (*arrow*).

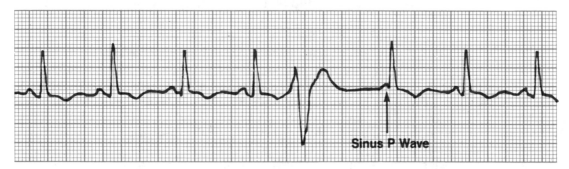

Sinus rhythm with one VPC followed by a junctional escape beat. The sinus P wave is partially inscribed in front of the junctional escape beat but bears no relationship to it.

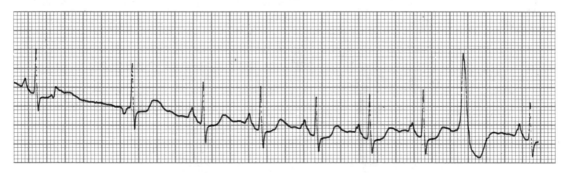

Sinus rhythm with a nonconducted APC followed by a pause terminated by a junctional escape beat. The junctional escape beat is preceded by an ectopic inverted P wave. One isolated VPC is also present.

ESCAPE BEATS AND RHYTHMS

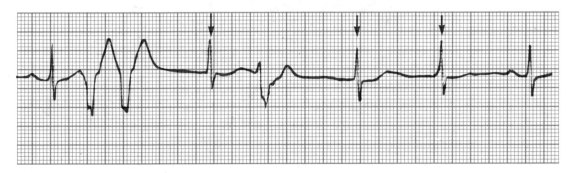

Sinus rhythm and first degree AV block and a pair of unifocal VPCs, the first one malignant. The VPCs are followed by a junctional escape beat, another VPC, and two more junctional escape beats (*arrows*), and sinus rhythm then resumes. The third junctional escape beat is preceded by the initial portion of a sinus P wave.

When a strip such as the one above is so filled with different arrhythmias, the only sensible way to approach the conglomeration is to eyeball the entire strip first. Get a feel for any regularity or pattern and try to pick out a sinus rhythm. The strip appears to have a regular rhythm other than three wide and bizarre beats that interrupt the rhythm. Take eyeball measurements of the PR and QRS to be sure that they are within the normal range. Then proceed from the first beat of the strip on the left and move slowly to the right, identifying each beat as you go. The PR interval is long, as seen with the first sinus beat, demonstrating first degree AV block, and the QRS interval is within normal range. The sinus beat is followed by two VPCs—the first of them malignant—which are in turn followed by a pause, which is normal. The pause is terminated by a beat without a PR interval—a junctional escape beat. That is followed by a multifocal VPC, which again is followed by an expected pause and is terminated with two junctional escape beats, and a return to sinus rhythm. This all sounds confusing, but if you follow the rhythm one beat at a time and move along the strip to the end, the identification of the arrhythmias becomes easier.

JUNCTIONAL ESCAPE RHYTHM

A junctional escape rhythm is a run of six or more junctional escape beats in a row at a rate below 60 beats per minute. This mechanism takes over as the heart rhythm when the sinus node fails to fire or when there is a blockage in the conduction system.

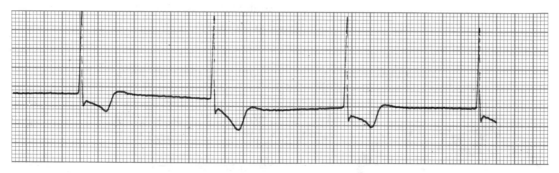

Junctional escape rhythm. No ectopic P waves are visible.

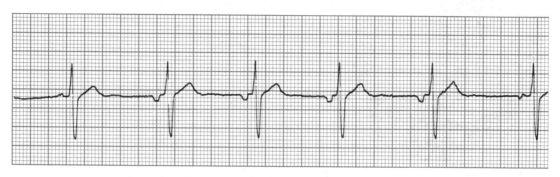

Junctional escape rhythm with inverted ectopic P waves preceding each QRS

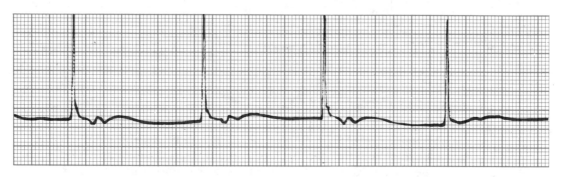

Junctional escape rhythm with inverted ectopic P waves following each QRS

ESCAPE BEATS AND RHYTHMS

VENTRICULAR ESCAPE BEAT

If a junctional escape beat does not terminate a pause in the heart, a ventricular escape beat will—it is hoped—come to the rescue. A focus in the ventricles fires and depolarizes the ventricle where it originates and then spreads with some delay through ventricular muscle to depolarize the other ventricle. Because of the delay in conduction through abnormal conduction pathways, a wide and bizarre-looking QRS is inscribed.

Ventricular escape beats can occur as isolated beats, or they can occur as pairs or in runs.

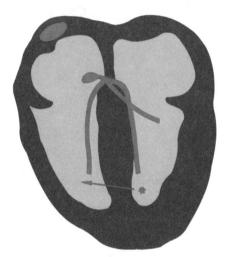

The following simplified criteria are used for recognition of a ventricular escape beat:

1. The ventricular escape beat is late in relation to the normal R-R cycle.
2. The QRS is wide and bizarre.

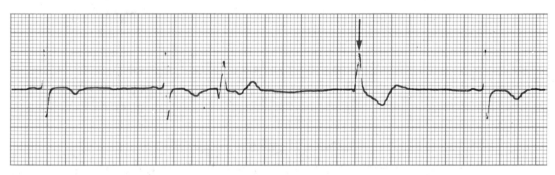

Sinus bradycardia with one VPC followed by a ventricular escape beat (*arrow*) and then back to sinus rhythm. The escape beat is not a second VPC because it does not arrive early but fires later than the normal R-R cycle.

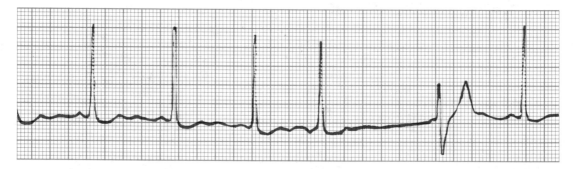

Sinus rhythm with a JPC and a probable nonconducted APC. The pause following the ectopic beats is terminated by a ventricular escape beat. The partially inscribed P wave before the escape beat is a sinus P wave but bears no relationship to the escape beat. The ventricular escape beat is late in relation to the normal R-R cycle.

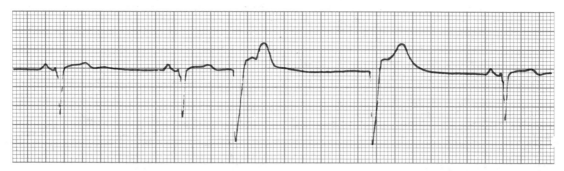

Sinus bradycardia with one VPC followed by a ventricular escape beat and back to sinus rhythm

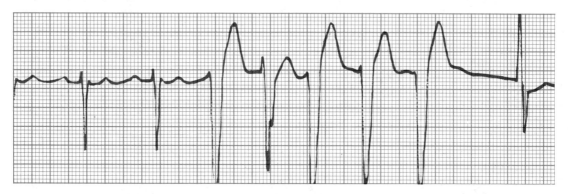

Sinus rhythm with five unifocal VPCs followed by a ventricular escape beat

VENTRICULAR ESCAPE RHYTHM

Six or more ventricular escape beats in a row at a rate below 40 beats per minute constitute a ventricular escape rhythm. This mechanism takes over as the heart rhythm when the sinus node fails to fire or when there is a blockage in the conduction system.

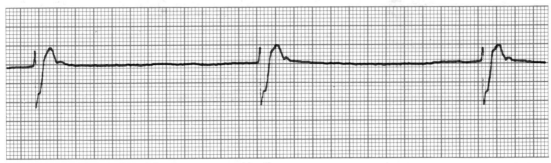

Ventricular escape rhythm

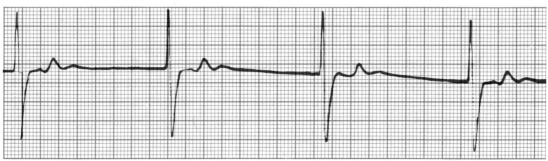

Ventricular escape rhythm

DIFFERENTIAL DIAGNOSIS

End diastolic VPC or ventricular escape beat?

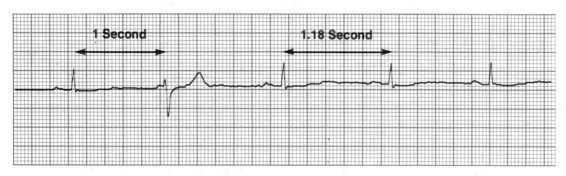

For the wide beat to be a ventricular escape beat it would have to be late in relation to the normal cardiac rhythm. The normal R-R cycle is 1.18 second, and the R-R interval of the questionable beat is shorter, at only 1 second. So it is not late in relation to the normal R-R cycle and not a ventricular escape beat but an end diastolic VPC coming immediately after a sinus P wave.

End diastolic VPC or ventricular escape beat?

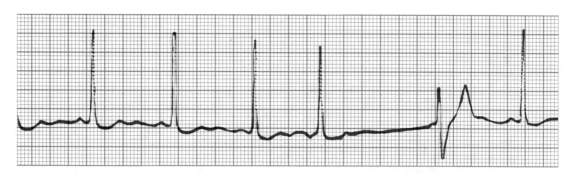

The wide and bizarre beat terminating the pause caused by a JPC and probable nonconducted APC is late in relation to the normal R-R cycle. This confirms the diagnosis of a ventricular escape beat rather than an end diastolic VPC occurring either slightly early or nearly on time with the normal R-R cycle.

Junctional escape beat or JPC?

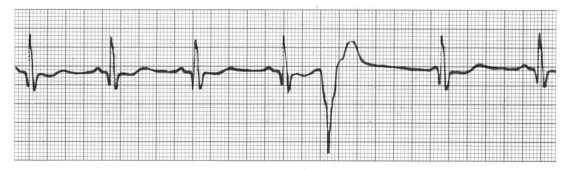

Sinus rhythm with bundle branch block with one malignant VPC.
The pause following the VPC is longer than the normal R-R cycle
and is terminated by a beat without a preceding sinus P wave.
Because the beat is late, a JPC is ruled out. A beat that is late, that
is preceded or followed by an inverted P wave or no visible P wave,
and that has a QRS complex resembling that of the normal cardiac
rhythm is a junctional escape beat.

PRACTICE ECG STRIPS

I have purposely included artifact in some of the ECG strips to simulate the types of strips you might expect to find in the field. Eyeball the PR and QRS intervals for normal or abnormal intervals rather than exact measurements. Then estimate the rate, identify the rhythm, and label any arrhythmias present.

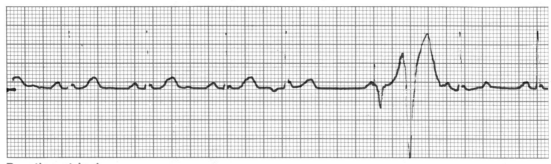

Practice strip 1

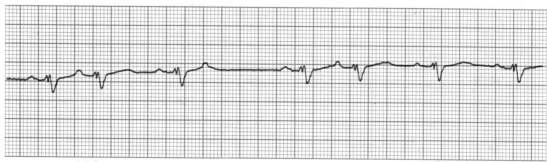

Practice strip 2

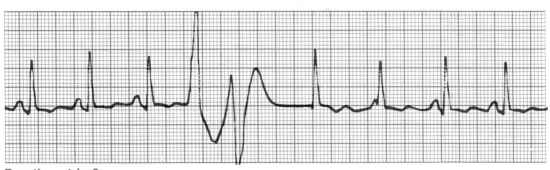

Practice strip 3

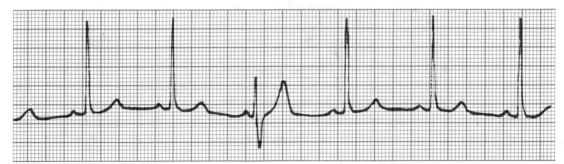

Practice strip 4

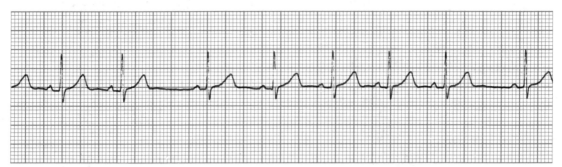

Practice strip 5

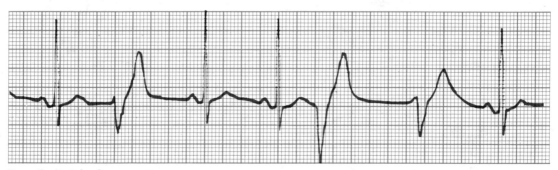

Practice strip 6

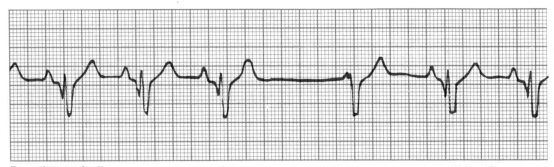

Practice strip 7

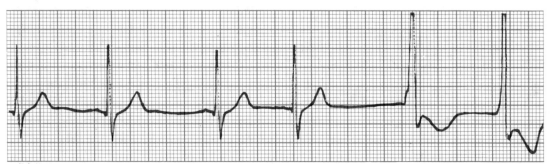

Practice strip 8

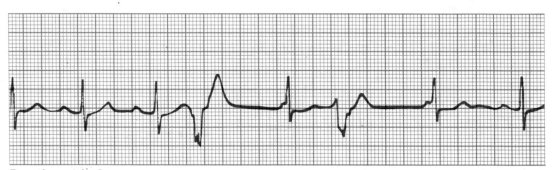

Practice strip 9

ESCAPE BEATS AND RHYTHMS

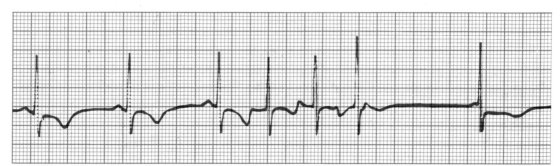

Practice strip 10

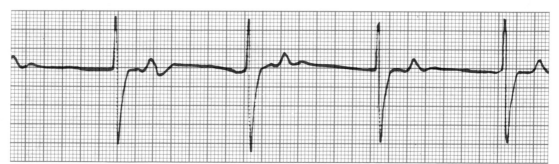

Practice strip 11

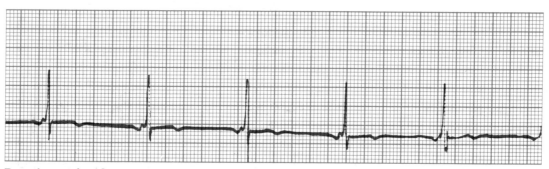

Practice strip 12

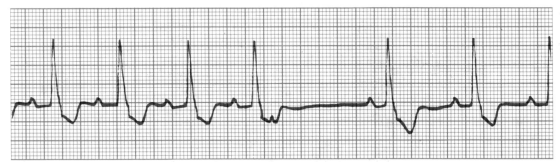

Practice strip 13

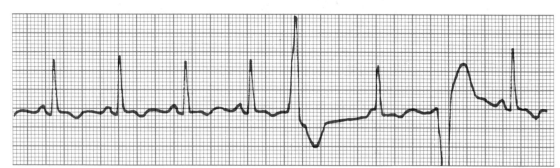

Practice strip 14

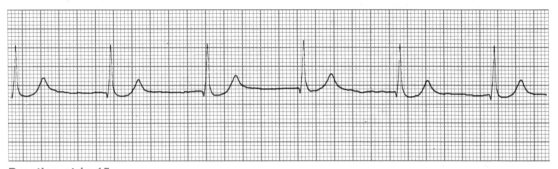

Practice strip 15

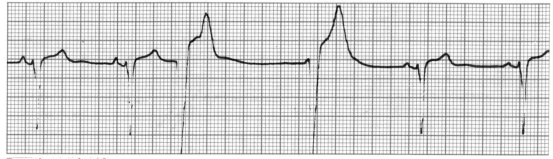

Practice strip 16

PRACTICE ECG STRIP ANSWERS

1. Sinus rhythm with one JPC followed by a ventricular escape beat and a malignant VPC and back to sinus rhythm

2. Sinus rhythm with two isolated APCs and one nonconducted APC

3. Sinus rhythm with a pair of multifocal VPCs followed by two junctional escape beats

4. Sinus rhythm with one end diastolic VPC

5. Sinus arrhythmia

6. Sinus rhythm with two unifocal VPCs, the second being followed by a ventricular escape beat

7. Sinus rhythm with bundle branch block and a nonconducted APC followed by a junctional escape beat

8. Sinus bradycardia with one JPC followed by two ventricular escape beats

9. Sinus rhythm with first degree AV block with two multifocal VPCs, the first being malignant, and each followed by a junctional escape beat

10. Sinus rhythm with four APCs in a row, the last being nonconducted, immediately followed by a junctional escape beat

11. Ventricular escape rhythm

12. Junctional escape rhythm

13. Sinus rhythm with first degree AV block, bundle branch block, and one nonconducted APC

14. Sinus rhythm with two multifocal VPCs, the first followed by a junctional escape beat

15. Junctional escape rhythm

16. Sinus bradycardia with a VPC followed by a ventricular escape beat

Chapter 7

SUPRAVENTRICULAR ECTOPIC RHYTHMS

Atrial and junctional rhythms are supraventricular rhythms and are less dangerous than the ventricular rhythms discussed in Chapter 8. It is often difficult to identify the heart rhythm when the heart rate is very rapid, so many examples will be given to help you acquire skill in rapid and accurate identification.

During monitoring, it is not always necessary to differentiate atrial from junctional tachycardia, but you must be able to differentiate between supraventricular and the more dangerous ventricular tachycardia.

ATRIAL RHYTHMS

Atrial ectopic rhythms are caused by rapid and repetitive firing of one or more ectopic foci located anywhere in the atria other than the sinus node. Although rates are given below for all the atrial rhythms, they are just a guide and are not ironclad rules.

Atrial Ectopic Rhythm Rates

Atrial tachycardia	140–220 per minute
Atrial tachycardia with block	140–220 per minute
Multifocal atrial tachycardia	100–200 per minute
Atrial flutter	220–350 per minute
Atrial fibrillation	350–650 per per minute

Atrial Tachycardia

A run of six or more unifocal APCs in a row constitutes atrial tachycardia. Often the term *paroxysmal atrial tachycardia (PAT)* is used, meaning a sudden burst of unifocal APCs. A focus in the atria, other than the SA node, depolarizes repeatedly and causes early, different-looking P waves. The remainder of depolarization occurs normally, and a QRS resembling that of the normal cardiac rhythm is usually recorded. The rate of atrial tachycardia is between 140 and 220 beats per minute and is usually regular.

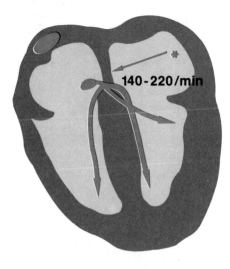

140-220/min

The following simplified criteria are used for recognition of atrial tachycardia:

1. Atrial trachycardia is composed of six or more APCs in a row with a regular P-P cycle between 140 and 220 beats per minute.
2. The QRS usually resembles that of a normal cardiac rhythm.

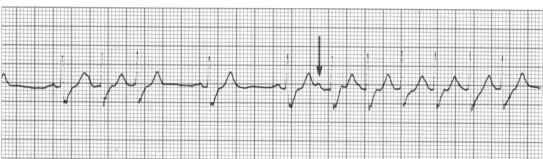

Sinus rhythm with a pair of APCs and a run of PAT. The arrow indicates the first ectopic P wave of the atrial tachycardia.

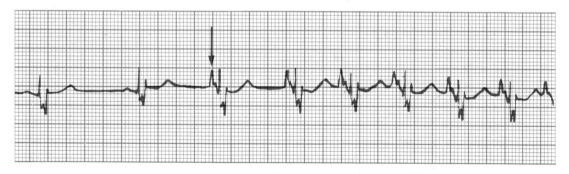

Sinus bradycardia with a run of PAT. The arrow indicates the first ectopic P wave of the tachycardia. The rate of the tachycardia is slow at first, and, as is often the case, it accelerates as the tachycardia continues. This is PAT with 1:1 conduction (one P wave for each QRS).

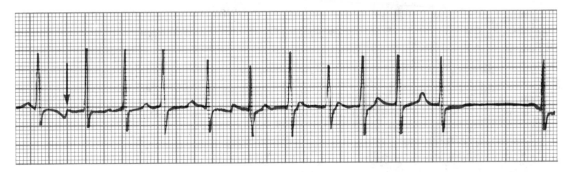

Sinus rhythm with a run of PAT and back to sinus rhythm. The arrow indicates the first ectopic P wave of the tachycardia.

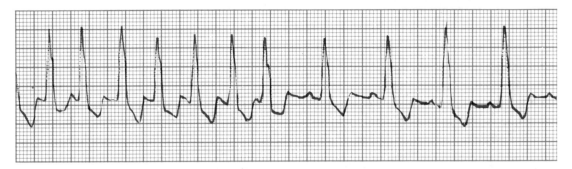

PAT at 150 per minute, reverting to sinus rhythm with bundle branch block. If the widened QRS complex of the sinus rhythm were not present to compare with the PAT, the run of PAT might be mistaken for a run of VPCs. Careful examination reveals ectopic P waves for each of the QRS complexes, confirming the diagnosis of PAT.

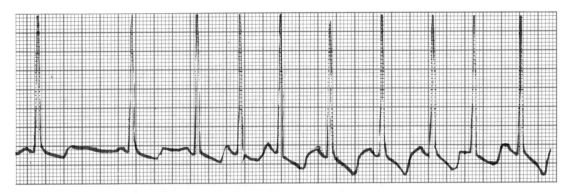

Sinus bradycardia with a run of PAT

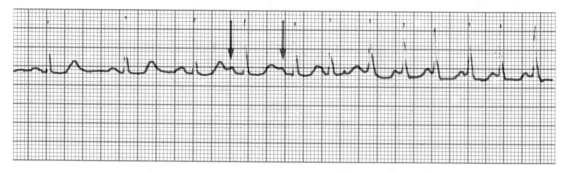

Sinus rhythm and a run of PAT. The first two beats of the tachycardia (*arrows*) display visible ectopic P waves and allow the diagnosis of PAT rather than the more general term *supraventricular tachycardia*.

Paroxysmal Atrial Tachycardia (PAT) With Block

If the rate of the atrial tachycardia is rapid, some of the ectopic P waves may find the AV node still refractory and recovering from the previous beat. Every ectopic P wave will not be conducted to the ventricles, and no QRS will occur. The P-P cycle is regular, but not all the P waves will be followed by QRS complexes. This lack of 1 : 1 conduction (one P wave for each QRS) in this arrhythmia actually prevents the heart from beating too rapidly by allowing only some of the P waves to conduct to the ventricles and produce a QRS complex.

The following simplified criteria are used for recognition of PAT with block:

1. PAT with block is a run of six or more APCs in a row with a regular P-P cycle between 140 and 200 beats per minute, but without all the ectopic P waves being conducted to the ventricles.
2. The QRS usually resembles that of a normal cardiac rhythm.

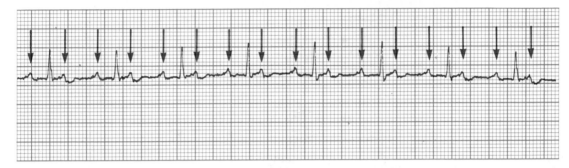

PAT with 2:1 block. The P-P cycle is regular at 150 per minute, and every other ectopic P wave is conducted to the ventricles, producing a ventricular rate of 75 per minute. Ectopic P waves are identified with an arrow. In all ECG strips, always examine T waves for the presence of possible hidden P waves.

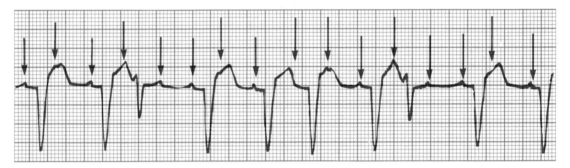

PAT with variable block and bundle branch block and two isolated VPCs. The atrial rate is regular at 150 beats per minute, and there is usually more than one P wave for each QRS. Ectopic P waves are labeled with arrows.

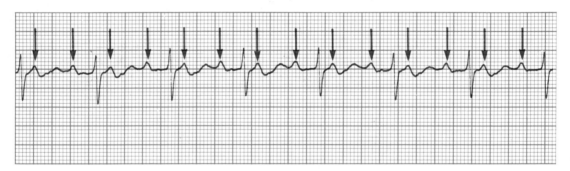

PAT with 2:1 block. The atrial rate is 150 beats per minute, and very other ectopic P wave is conducted to the ventricles, producing a ventricular rate of 75 per minute. Ectopic P waves are identified with arrows.

HOW TO QUICKLY AND ACCURATELY MASTER ARRHYTHMIA INTERPRETATION

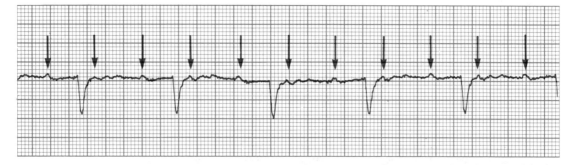

PAT with 2:1 block. The atrial rate is 120 beats per minute, and every other ectopic P wave is conducted to the ventricles, producing a ventricular rate of 60 beats per minute. Ectopic P waves are identified with arrows. In this strip, discovering the second ectopic P wave for each QRS is more difficult—but possible. Careful examination of each PQRST wave is mandatory.

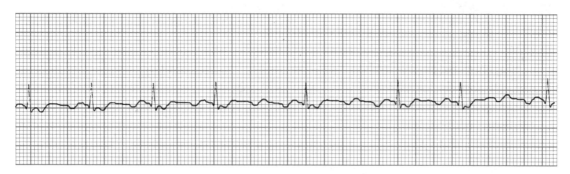

The ectopic P waves are more apparent as inverted P waves. The P-P cycle is regular at 170 beats per minute, and every second or third P wave is followed by a QRS. This is PAT with 2:1 and 3:1 block.

Multifocal Atrial Tachycardia

A run of six or more multifocal APCs in a row constitutes a multifocal atrial tachycardia. Because there is more than one ectopic atrial focus, the P waves vary in configuration, the PR intervals do not remain constant, and the P-P cycles are irregular. Some nonconducted APCs may occur.

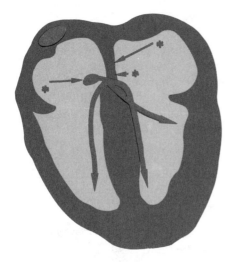

The following simplified criteria are used for recognition of multifocal atrial tachycardia:

1. Multifocal atrial tachycardia is composed of six or more multifocal APCs in a row with an irregular P-P cycle between 100 and 200 beats per minute.

2. The P waves vary in configuration, and the PR intervals vary in duration.

3. The QRS usually resembles that of a normal cardiac rhythm.

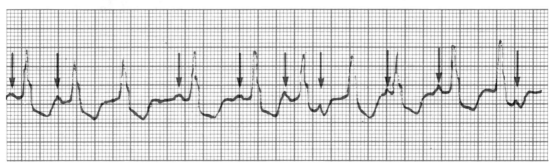

Multifocal atrial tachycardia with different P wave configurations, varying PR intervals, and an irregular rate. Visible ectopic P waves are labeled with arrows.

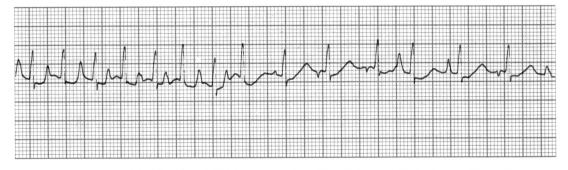

Multifocal atrial tachycardia with different P wave configurations, varying PR intervals, and an irregular rate

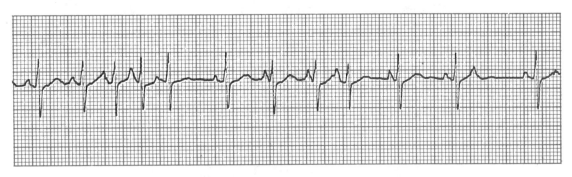

Notice the different P wave configurations and varying PR intervals of the multifocal atrial tachycardia. There is a nonconducted APC at the end of the strip, and the P-P cycle throughout the strip is irregular, as expected.

Atrial Flutter

One theory of impulse formation in atrial flutter is a repetitive firing of one focus in the atria between 220 and 350 per minute. Because the atrial rate is so rapid, flutter (*F*) waves replace the P waves on the ECG, take on a characteristic sawtooth configuration, and often distort the ST and T waves on the ECG strip. Most often, not all the flutter waves are able to conduct to the ventricles because the AV node remains refractory from previous beats. The usual lack of 1:1 conduction in this arrhythmia actually prevents the heart from beating too rapidly by allowing only some of the F waves to conduct to the ventricles and produce a QRS complex. One of the dangers of atrial flutter is that all the F waves occurring may be conducted to the ventricles—1:1 conduction—causing a heart rhythm between 220 and 350 per minute and compromising the circulatory system.

The ventricles usually respond to the even-numbered waves—second, producing 2:1 conduction; fourth, producing 4:1 conduction, and so on—or may respond sporadically at various conduction ratios.

FLUTTER WAVES

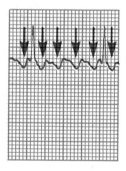

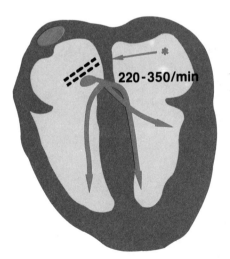

220-350/min

The following simplified criteria are used for recognition of atrial flutter:

1. Atrial flutter is the repetitive firing of one focus in the atria with a regular F-F cycle at 220 to 350 per minute.
2. F waves replace P waves.
3. The QRS usually resembles that of a normal cardiac rhythm.

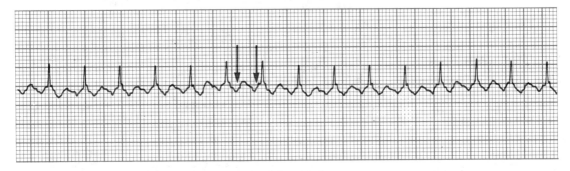

Atrial flutter at 300 beats per minute with 2:1 conduction and a ventricular response of 150. The ventricles respond to every other flutter wave. The flutter waves deform the ST-T segments of the QRS complexes. Two flutter waves are marked with arrows.

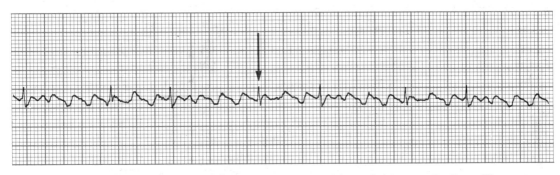

Atrial flutter at 300 per minute with variable conduction. The ventricles randomly respond to the flutter waves. The QRS complexes are small and are almost camouflaged by the flutter waves. One QRS complex is labeled (*arrow*); notice how the flutter waves distort its ST segment and T wave.

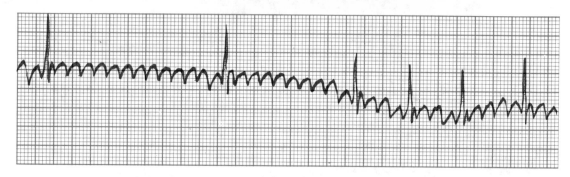

Atrial flutter with variable conduction and a slow ventricular response. The long ventricular pauses sometimes seen in atrial flutter represent a blockage or delay in conduction below the atria and can cause loss of cerebral function.

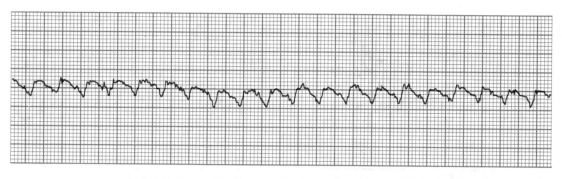

Atrial flutter at 220 per minute with 1:1 conduction. The danger of every flutter wave conducting through the AV node to the ventricles is the very rapid and dangerous ventricular rates that can occur. Fortunately, the flutter rate in this patient is not the usual 300 beats per minute, or the ventricular response in this 1:1 conduction would compromise the circulatory system.

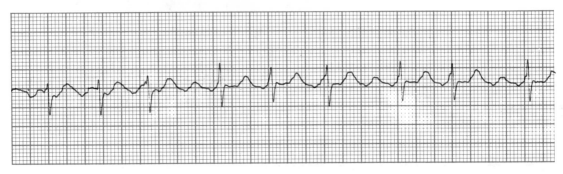

Atrial flutter at 220 per minute with variable block. The flutter waves may at times resemble P waves rather than F waves, but the atrial rate of 220 or greater distinguishes flutter waves from P waves.

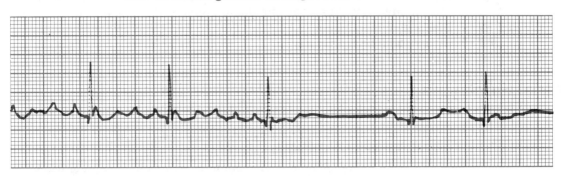

Atrial flutter at 300 beats per minute with variable conduction and conversion to sinus rhythm with first degree AV block and one isolated APC.

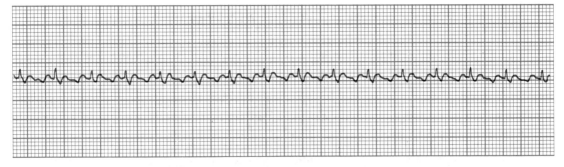

Atrial flutter at 300 beats per minute with 2:1 conduction. If you look quickly, you might mistake this for sinus tachycardia at 150 beats per minute rather than atrial flutter. Always be alert for the possibility of the hidden ectopic atrial wave in the preceding ST or T wave. When the ventricular rate is 150 beats per minute, always suspect atrial flutter with 2:1 conduction and look for the additional flutter wave.

SUPRAVENTRICULAR ECTOPIC RHYTHMS

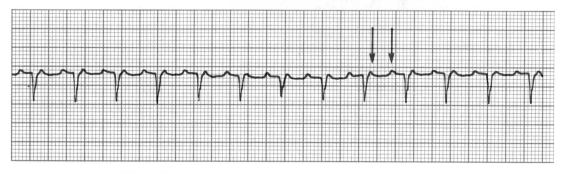

Atrial flutter with 2:1 conduction. Two F waves are labeled with arrows to make identification easier. Although these F waves appear to be P waves, the atrial rate of 250 confirms atrial flutter. The hidden F waves have the same configuration as the obvious ones, and they occur exactly on time to make the F-F cycle regular at 250 beats per minute.

Atrial Fibrillation

One theory of impulse formation in atrial fibrillation is that there are multiple ectopic foci in the atria firing repetitively at a rate of 350 to 650 beats per minute. One ectopic focus fires immediately after another, causing the atria to quiver continuously rather than contract. These fibrillatory (f) waves occurring so rapidly make it difficult to determine the atrial rate. Fibrillatory waves are divided into two categories, coarse and fine.

FIBRILLATORY WAVES

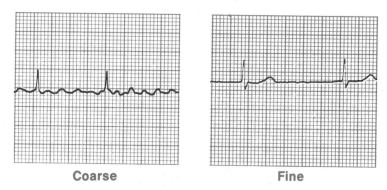

| Coarse | Fine |

Only some of the f waves can intermittently be conducted through the AV node to the ventricles because the AV node is constantly rendered refractory by the multiple fibrillatory impulses. This produces the characteristic irregular ventricular rate of atrial fibrillation. If the ventricular rate is extremely high, this irregularity is often difficult to see, and the diagnosis of atrial tachycardia may mistakenly be made. Slow ventricular rates, because of blockage or delay in the conduction system below the atria, can compromise the circulatory system.

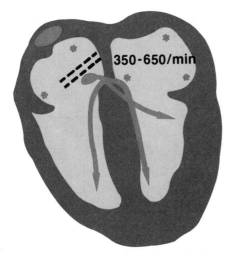

The following simplified criteria are used for recognition of atrial fibrillation:

1. Multifocal f waves replace P waves at a rate of 350 to 650 beats per minute.

2. Irregular ventricular response (R-R cycle constantly varying). If the ventricular rate is rapid, irregularity is more difficult to determine.

3. The QRS usually resembles that of a normal cardiac rhythm.

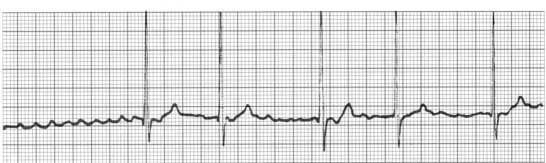

Atrial fibrillation with the characteristic irregular ventricular response

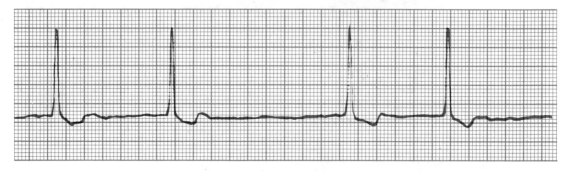

Atrial fibrillation with a slow ventricular response and no escape beats terminating long R-R cycles

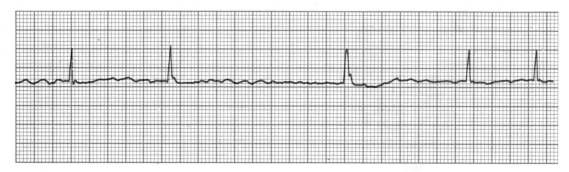

Atrial fibrillation with a slow ventricular response and a ventricular escape beat rescuing the heat during a long ventricular pause

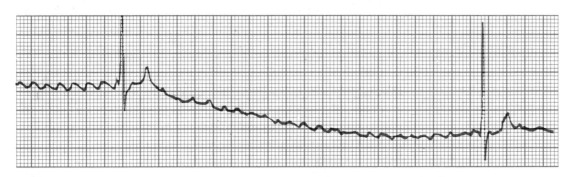

Atrial fibrillation with a dangerous four-second pause and no escape mechanism evident to rescue the heart

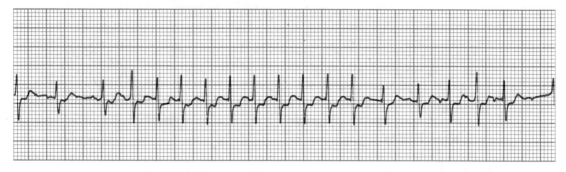

Atrial fibrillation with a very rapid ventricular response simulating a fast, regular ventricular rhythm

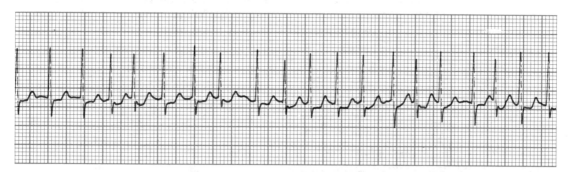

Atrial fibrillation with a rapid ventricular response simulating regularity of rhythm. Although no coarse fibrillatory waves can be identified, the irregular ventricular response is sufficient evidence for the diagnosis of atrial fibrillation.

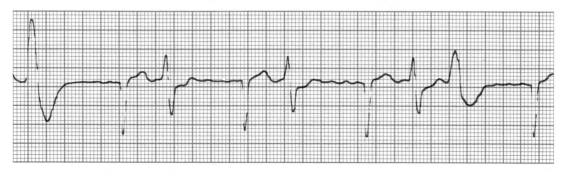

Atrial fibrillation with isolated multifocal VPCs and one pair. There are no P waves, and the R-R cycle is irregular. Coarse fibrillatory waves are visible between the QRS complexes.

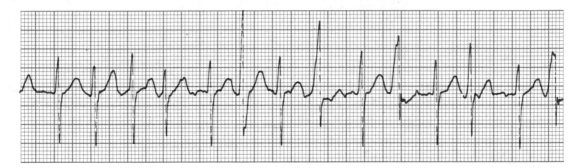

Atrial fibrillation with a rapid ventricular response and four isolated multifocal VPCs. The ventricular rate appears almost regular, but on closer examination it reveals that the definite ventricular irregularity of atrial fibrillation does indeed exist. Without evidence of P waves the diagnosis of atrial fibrillation is most logical.

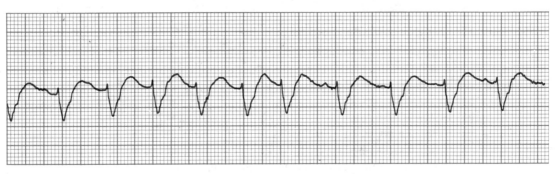

Atrial fibrillation with a bundle branch block. The irregular ventricular response is the clue to atrial fibrillation. A first impression for the strip could easily be a run of VPCs, but the irregular ventricular response and the presence of fine fibrillatory waves rule it out.

JUNCTIONAL RHYTHMS

Junctional ectopic rhythms are caused by repetitive and rapid firing of an ectopic focus located in or surrounding the AV node.

Junctional Ectopic Rhythm Rates

Accelerated junctional rhythm   60–99 beats per minute

Junctional tachycardia   100–220 beats per minute

Accelerated Junctional Rhythm and Junctional Tachycardia

Rapid and repetitive firing of six or more JPCs in a row constitutes an accelerated junctional rhythm or junctional tachycardia, depending on the rate. A focus in or around the AV node depolarizes repeatedly and causes early, inverted P waves. Then there are two scenarios: (1) either inverted P waves precede or follow the QRS complexes, or (2) no P waves will be visible. The remainder of depolarization occurs normally, and a QRS resembling that of the normal cardiac rhythm is usually recorded. The rate is usually regular, between 60 and 99 beats per minute for an accelerated junctional rhythm and between 100 and 220 for a junctional tachycardia.

During a slower junctional rhythm, the sinus node may continue to fire independent of the junctional rhythm and almost at the same rate. This is called *AV dissociation* and represents a dual rhythm in which the atria and ventricles beat independently, each under the control of a separate pacemaking focus and each temporarily prevented from depolarizing the other and rendering it refractory. Intermittently, the sinus P wave floats in and out of the QRS complex but bears no relationship to it. The junctional rhythm is the important arrhythmia; intermittent AV dissociation is incidental.

The following simplified criteria are used for recognition of accelerated junctional rhythm and junctional tachycardia:

1. Six or more JPCs occur in a row.
2. The QRS usually resembles that of a normal cardiac rhythm.
3. The ventricular rate is between 60 and 99 beats per minute for an accelerated junctional rhythm and between 100 and 220 beats per minute for a junctional tachycardia.

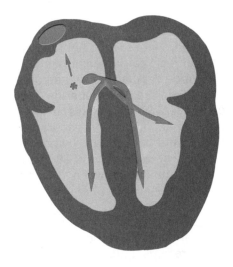

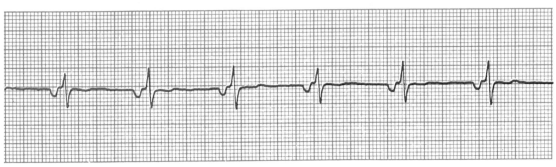

Accelerated junctional rhythm with inverted P waves preceding each QRS

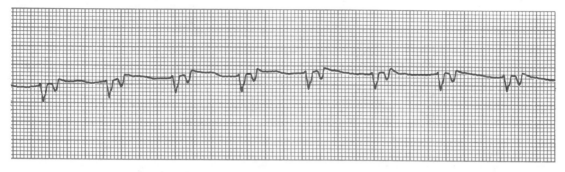

Accelerated junctional rhythm with inverted P waves following each QRS

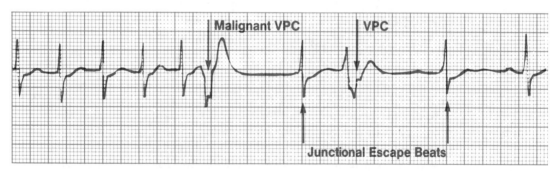

Junctional tachycardia with no ectopic P waves visible

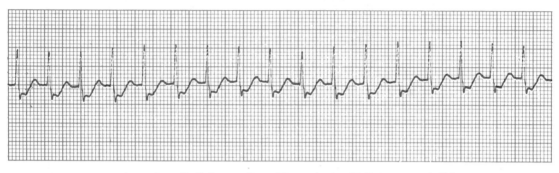

Junctional tachycardia with two multifocal VPCs, the first malignant. Each pause following the VPCs is terminated by a junctional escape beat, and then sinus rhythm with first degree AV block occurs. The first five beats of the strip show no apparent P waves and a regular R-R cycle, which rules in favor of junctional tachycardia rather than atrial fibrillation. The malignant VPC terminates the junctional tachycardia, and a pause is then terminated by a junctional escape beat with the beginning of a sinus P wave preceding it. Another VPC is recorded, followed by another junctional escape beat. Then the heart begins sinus rhythm with first degree AV block.

SUPRAVENTRICULAR ECTOPIC RHYTHMS

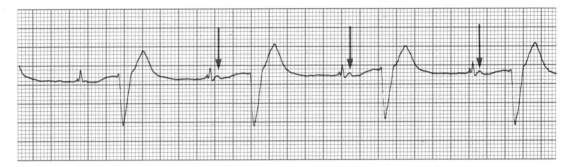

Accelerated junctional rhythm with unifocal VPCs in bigeminy. The first beat of the strip and every other beat thereafter shows no sinus P wave preceding the QRS. The beats occur in a regular rhythm interrupted by VPCs in bigeminy. If you look directly after the QRS complexes of the junctional rhythm, you will see upright sinus P waves (*arrows*). AV dissociation is present, with the junctional tachycardia controlling the ventricles, and the atria are under the control of sinus rhythm. The rates are almost identical but are temporarily functioning independently.

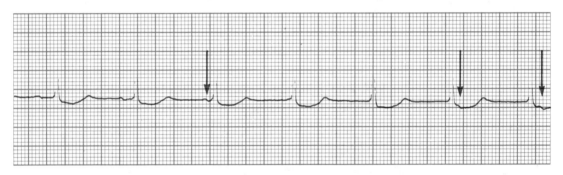

Sinus rhythm is recorded for the first two beats, and then AV dissociation occurs as the sinus P wave floats into the QRS complex. An accelerated junctional rhythm takes control of the ventricles, and the atria are under the control of the sinus rhythm. The visible sinus P waves occurring during the AV dissociation are labeled with arrows.

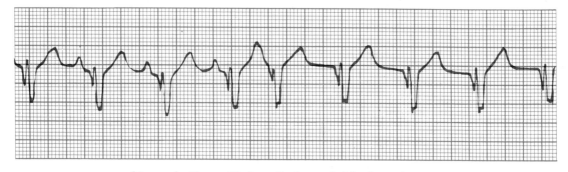

Sinus rhythm with bundle branch block and one isolated APC
followed by a run of accelerated junctional rhythm

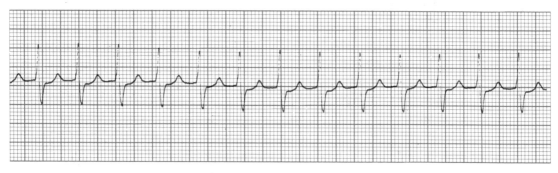

Junctional tachycardia with no ectopic P waves visible

SUPRAVENTRICULAR ECTOPIC RHYTHMS

SUPRAVENTRICULAR TACHYCARDIA

When it is impossible to differentiate between atrial and junctional tachycardia and make a specific diagnosis, it is permissible to use the term *supraventricular tachycardia*. It is often difficult to make an accurate identification of an arrhythmia when the rate is high or when artifact is present. Accurate identification of supraventricular tachycardia versus ventricular tachycardia is the primary concern.

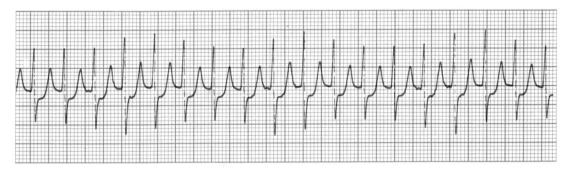

It is impossible to tell whether this strip represents junctional tachycardia with no ectopic P waves or atrial tachycardia with ectopic P waves superimposed on T waves. The interpretation of supraventricular tachycardia at 180 beats per minute is correct.

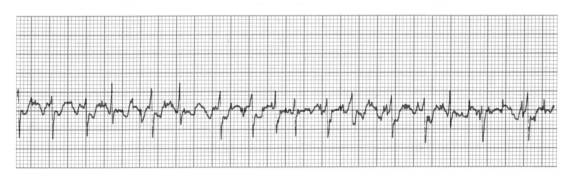

Is this atrial flutter with variable block, atrial fibrillation, or multifocal atrial tachycardia? Because of the artifact it is impossible to make a distinction, and it is sufficient to diagnose supraventricular tachycardia with a ventricular rate of approximately 170 beats per minute.

DIFFERENTIAL DIAGNOSIS

Junctional tachycardia or sinus rhythm with first degree AV block?

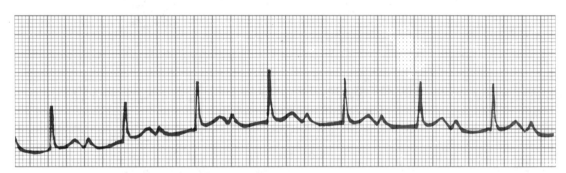

Initially this strip appears to be an accelerated junctional rhythm, but further examination reveals that the T wave is disfigured by the P wave of sinus rhythm and first degree AV block. T waves do not take on an M shape unless they are distorted by P waves.

Junctional tachycardia or atrial flutter?

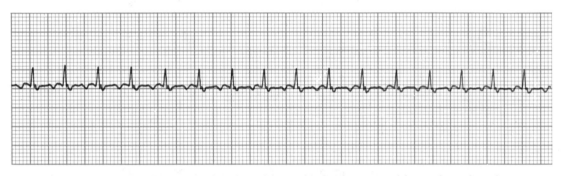

On first examination this arrhythmia resembles a junctional tachycardia because of the apparent inverted P waves preceding each QRS complex. On closer inspection, however, there are two flutter waves for each QRS appearing at a regular rate of 330 beats per minute. The second flutter wave is buried in the T wave of the previous QRS, and this confirms the diagnosis of atrial flutter with 2:1 block.

Junctional tachycardia or atrial flutter?

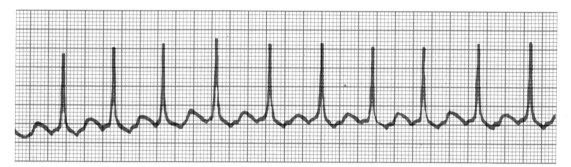

There is a definite characteristic sawtooth configuration
representing flutter waves. There should be no problem in
identifying them in this strip. Although there appear to be inverted P
waves preceding each QRS, the second flutter wave for each QRS
is visible and is buried in the ST segment of the previous beat.

Junctional tachycardia or atrial flutter?

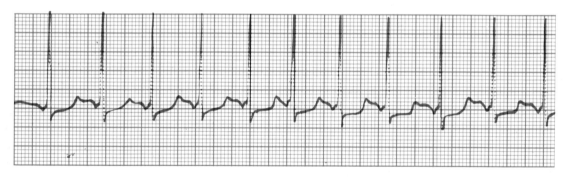

There are clear inverted P waves preceding each QRS complex but
no visible evidence of additional P waves buried in the T waves.
None of the ST segments or T waves are distorted with ectopic
waves, confirming the diagnosis of junctional tachycardia.

PAT or atrial flutter?

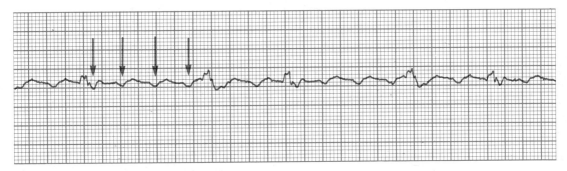

The four waves labeled with arrows appear to be flutter waves. But the atrial rate of 170 beats per minute rules out atrial flutter in favor of PAT with variable block.

Atrial fibrillation or multifocal atrial tachycardia?

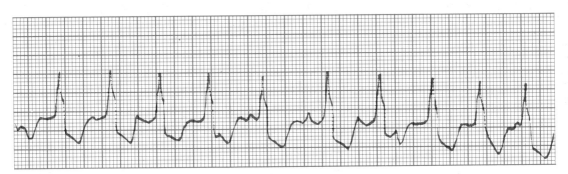

The ventricular rate is irregular, suggesting atrial fibrillation. But on close inspection, multiple P waves with varying PR intervals are evident, confirming the diagnosis of multifocal atrial tachycardia.

PAT with 2 : 1 block or nonconducted APCs in bigeminy?

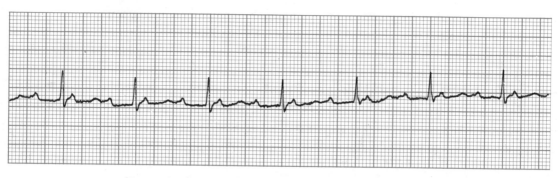

Sinus rhythm with first degree AV block is clearly visible. On close
examination an additional P wave is seen in each previous T wave,
leading one to suspect either nonconducted APCs or PAT with 2 : 1
block. The P-P cycle is regular, with no early P waves, ruling out
nonconducted APCs and confirming PAT with 2 : 1 block.

PRACTICE ECG STRIPS

I have purposely included artifact in some of the ECG strips to simulate the types of strips you might expect to find in the field. Eyeball
the PR and QRS intervals for normal or abnormal intervals rather
than exact measurements. Then estimate the rate, identify the rhythm,
and label any arrhythmias present.

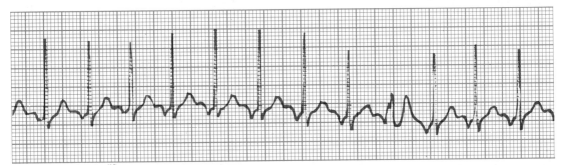

Practice strip 1

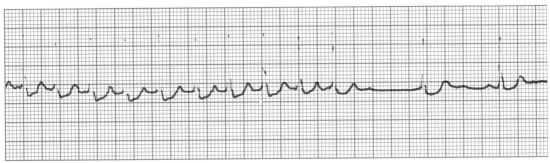

Practice strip 2

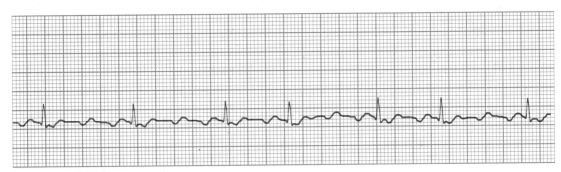

Practice strip 3

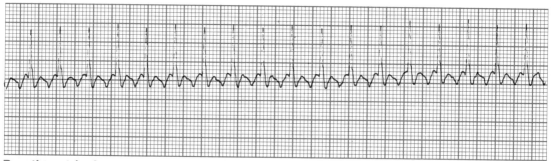

Practice strip 4

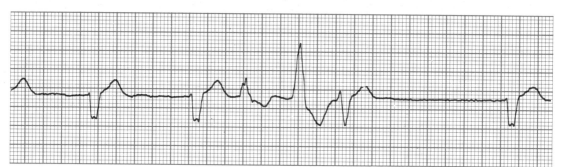

Practice strip 5

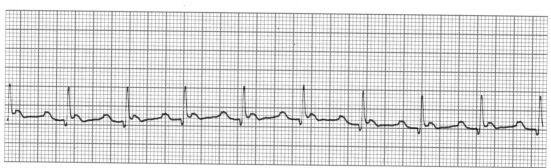

Practice strip 6

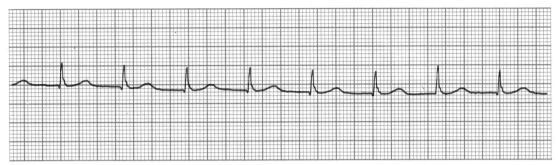

Practice strip 7

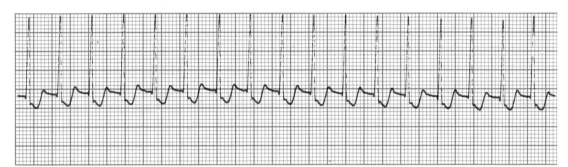

Practice strip 8

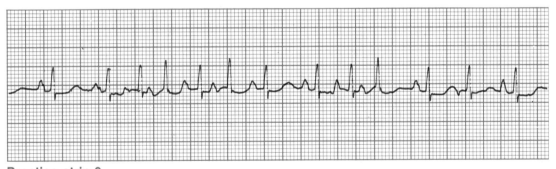

Practice strip 9

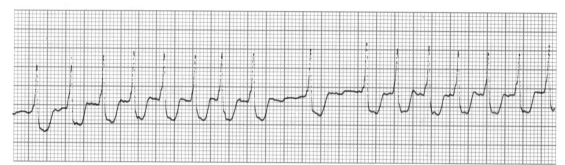

Practice strip 10

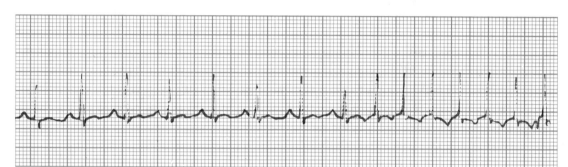

Practice strip 11

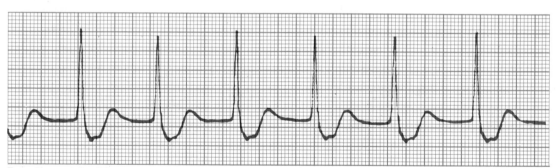

Practice strip 12

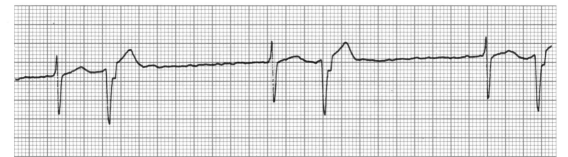

Practice strip 13

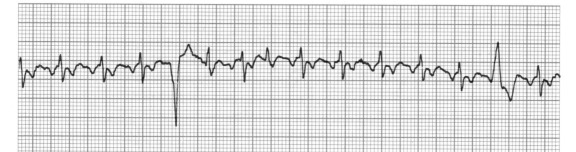

Practice strip 14

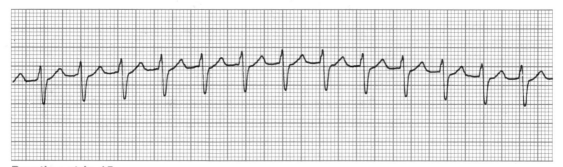

Practice strip 15

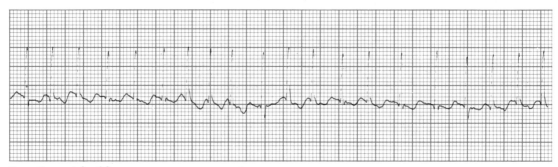

Practice strip 16

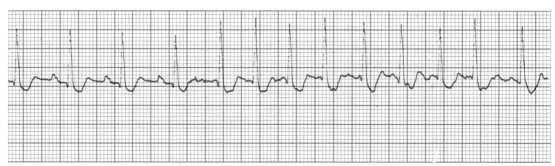

Practice strip 17

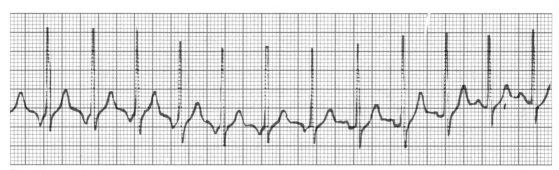

Practice strip 18

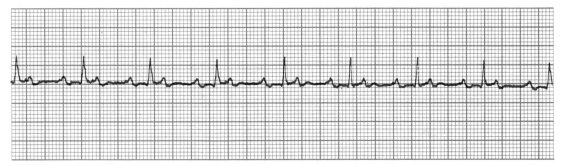

Practice strip 19

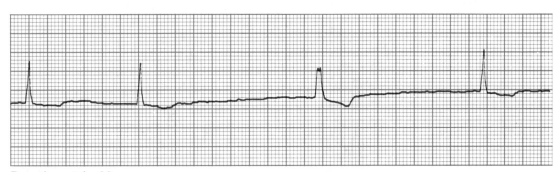

Practice strip 20

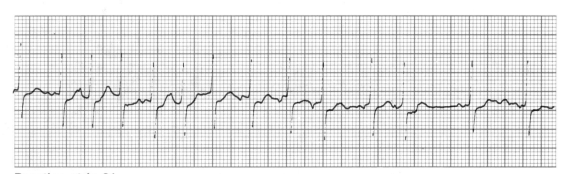

Practice strip 21

SUPRAVENTRICULAR ECTOPIC RHYTHMS

131

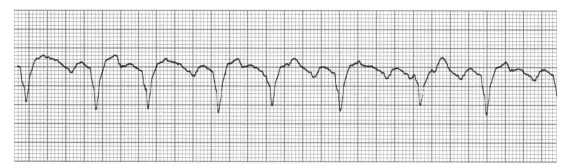

Practice strip 22

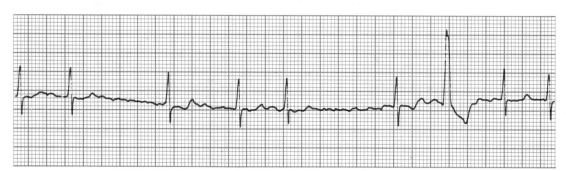

Practice strip 23

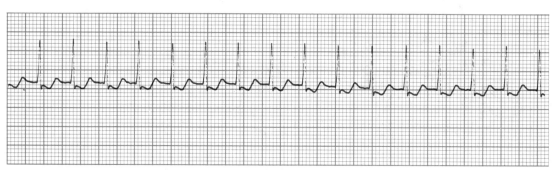

Practice strip 24

PRACTICE ECG STRIP ANSWERS

1. Junctional tachycardia with one VPC
2. Atrial tachycardia terminated by a junctional escape beat and then sinus rhythm
3. PAT with variable block
4. Atrial flutter with 2:1 block
5. Atrial fibrillation with bundle branch block and three multifocal VPCs in a row
6. PAT with 2:1 block
7. Accelerated junctional rhythm
8. Supraventricular tachycardia
9. Multifocal atrial tachycardia
10. Atrial fibrillation
11. Sinus tachycardia converting to junctional tachycardia
12. Accelerated junctional rhythm
13. Atrial fibrillation with unifocal VPCs in bigeminy
14. Atrial flutter with 2:1 block and two isolated multifocal VPCs
15. Junctional tachycardia
16. Atrial fibrillation
17. Sinus tachycardia converting to atrial fibrillation
18. Junctional tachycardia converting to sinus tachycardia
19. PAT with 2:1 block
20. Atrial fibrillation with a slow ventricular rate and one ventricular escape beat
21. Atrial fibrillation
22. Atrial flutter with varying block and bundle branch block
23. Atrial fibrillation with one isolated VPC
24. Supraventricular tachycardia

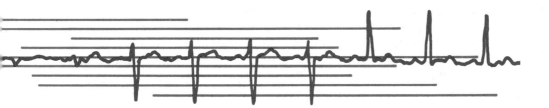

Chapter 8

VENTRICULAR ECTOPIC RHYTHMS

Ventricular ectopic rhythms are caused by repetitive firing of one or more ectopic foci located in the ventricles. These rhythms are an emergency and must be diagnosed immediately. Care must be used to accurately differentiate the ventricular from the supraventricular rhythms.

Ventricular Ectopic Rhythm Rates

Accelerated idioventricular rhythm	40–99 per minute
Ventricular tachycardia	100–250 per minute
Ventricular flutter	150–300 per minute
Ventricular fibrillation	150–500 per minute

ACCELERATED IDIOVENTRICULAR RHYTHM

An accelerated idioventricular rhythm is a repetitive firing of a focus in the ventricles at a rate of 40 to 99 beats per minute. A focus in one ventricle fires and depolarizes the ventricle where it originates, and the depolarization spreads, with delay, through ventricular muscle to depolarize the other ventricle. Because of the delay in conduction through abnormal conduction pathways, wide and bizarre-looking QRS complexes are inscribed.

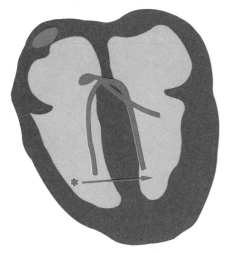

The following simplified criteria are used for recognition of an accelerated idioventricular rhythm:

1. Accelerated idioventricular rhythm is the repetitive firing of a focus in the ventricles at a regular rate of 40 to 99 beats per minute.
2. QRS complexes are wide and bizarre.
3. No ectopic P waves are present.

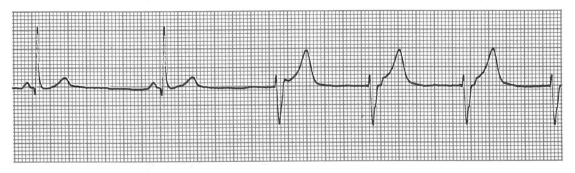

Sinus bradycardia followed by a run of accelerated idioventricular rhythm

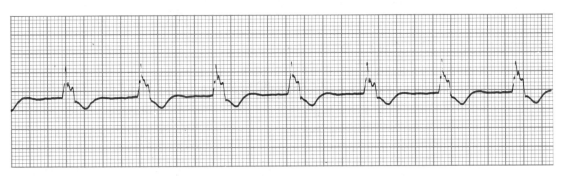

Accelerated idioventricular rhythm at 70 beats per minute. There is no evidence of P-wave activity, and the QRS is wide and bizarre.

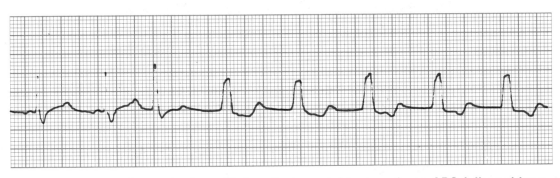

Sinus rhythm with bundle branch block and one APC followed by a run of accelerated idioventricular rhythm.

VENTRICULAR ECTOPIC RHYTHMS

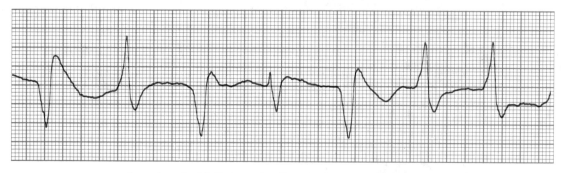

Accelerated idioventricular rhythm of multifocal origin. The rate is regular but represents a ventricular rhythm from more than one focus. No atrial activity is noted.

VENTRICULAR TACHYCARDIA

Ventricular tachycardia is a rapid and repetitive firing of six or more VPCs in a row. A focus in one ventricle fires and depolarizes the ventricle where it originates, and the depolarization spreads, with delay, through ventricular muscle to depolarize the other ventricle. Because of the delay in conduction through abnormal conduction pathways, wide, bizarre-looking QRS complexes are inscribed. The resulting wide QRS complexes have no corresponding ectopic P waves.

When the ventricles depolarize and contract rapidly with this arrhythmia, the volume of blood ejected into the circulation is often inadequate. This arrhythmia must be diagnosed immediately: ventricular tachycardia is an emergency. If left untreated, it often degenerates into ventricular flutter or fibrillation.

If the heart is in sinus rhythm, the sinus cycle may continue to fire completely independent of the ventricular tachycardia. This is called *AV dissociation* and is a dual rhythm in which the atria and ventricles beat independently, each under the control of a separate pacemaking focus. Ventricular tachycardia is the critical arrhythmia; AV dissociation is incidental.

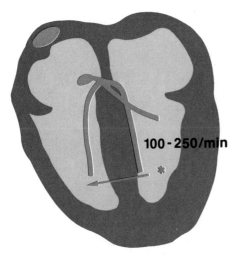

100 - 250/min

The following simple criteria are used for recognition of ventricular tachycardia:

1. A run of six or more VPCs occurs at a rate between 100 and 250 beats per minute.

2. QRS complexes are wide and bizarre.

3. No ectopic P waves are present. If the heart rate is sinus, the sinus P waves usually continue with their cycle, unaffected by the tachycardia, demonstrating AV dissociation.

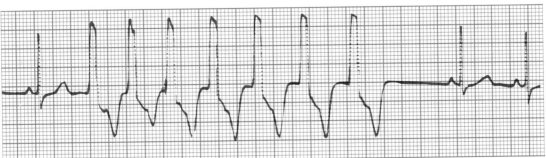

Sinus rhythm with a run of ventricular tachycardia and a spontaneous conversion back to sinus rhythm

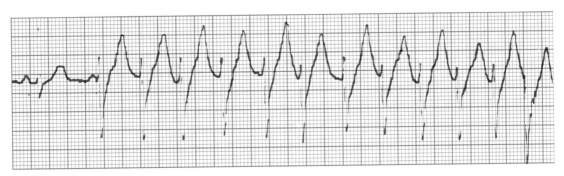

Sinus rhythm with a run of ventricular tachycardia beginning with an end diastolic VPC

VENTRICULAR ECTOPIC RHYTHMS

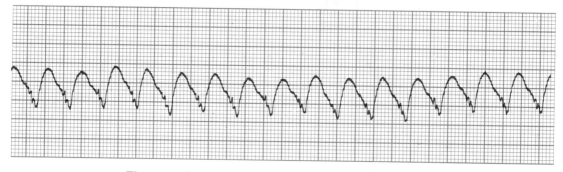

The ventricular tachycardia presented in this strip eventually progressed to ventricular fibrillation and the death of the patient.

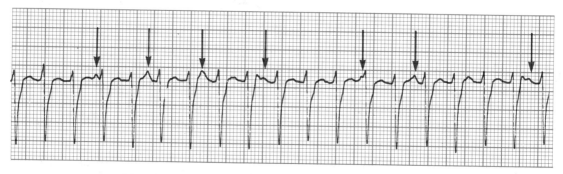

Sinus rhythm with a run of ventricular tachycardia, which progressed to ventricular fibrillation and eventual death of the patient.

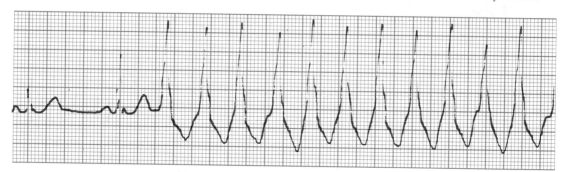

Ventricular tachycardia at 190 per minute with sinus P waves occurring at a rate of 100 per minute, demonstrating AV dissociation. Visible sinus P waves are labeled (*arrows*). The atria and ventricles are each under the control of a separate pacemaking focus and have no correlation with each other. The important diagnosis is ventricular tachycardia; the AV dissociation is incidental.

HOW TO QUICKLY AND ACCURATELY MASTER ARRHYTHMIA INTERPRETATION

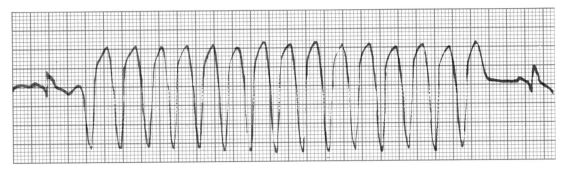

Sinus rhythm with a run of ventricular tachycardia and spontaneous conversion back to sinus rhythm

VENTRICULAR FLUTTER

In ventricular flutter there is a rapid and repetitive firing of one or more ventricular ectopic foci at a rate of 150 to 300 per minute. No atrial activity can be recognized, and the QRS complexes appear to run into each other with no visible ST segments or T waves. Ventricular flutter is an emergency.

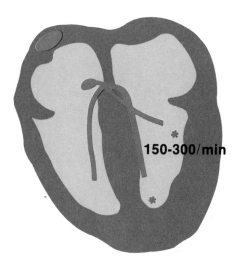

150-300/min

The following simplified criteria are used for recognition of ventricular flutter:

1. The QRS complexes appear to run into each other with no visible ST segments or T waves at a rate between 150 and 300 beats per minute.
2. No atrial activity can be recognized.

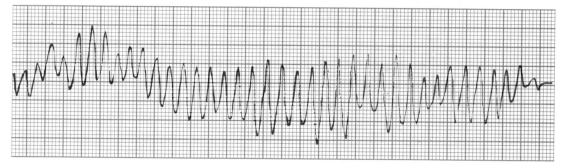

Ventricular flutter

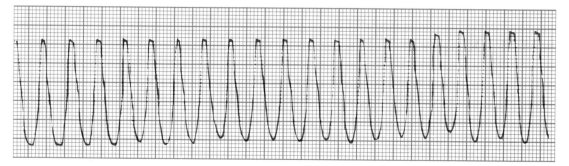

Ventricular flutter

VENTRICULAR FIBRILLATION

Multiple ventricular foci rapidly and repetitively fire at random 150 to 500 times per minute. This produces no recognizable QRS complexes or atrial activity on the ECG recording. Virtually no blood is ejected into the systemic circulation, and death will occur if no corrective action is taken. Because of its characteristic appearance, no other arrhythmia can be confused with ventricular fibrillation.

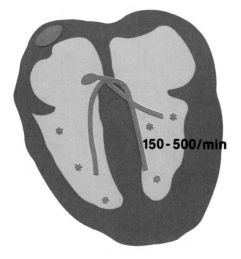

150-500/min

The following simplified criteria are used for recognition of ventricular fibrillation:

1. No atrial activity or QRS complexes can be recognized.
2. The rhythm is extremely irregular.

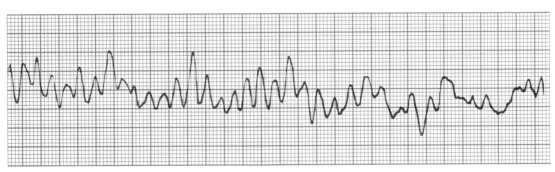

Coarse ventricular fibrillation

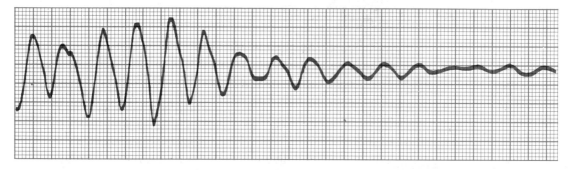

Coarse ventricular fibrillation progressing to fine ventricular fibrillation

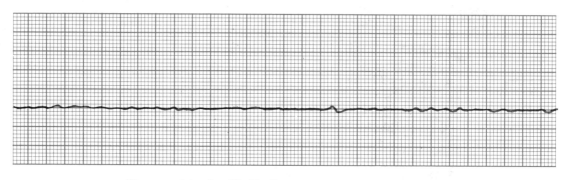

Fine ventricular fibrillation

DIFFERENTIAL DIAGNOSIS

Ventricular tachycardia or sinus tachycardia with bundle branch block?

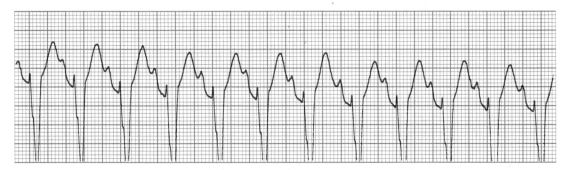

At first glance an identification of ventricular tachycardia is almost certain. But sinus P waves preceding each QRS and having a constant PR interval are discovered. The widened QRS is due to a bundle branch block.

Ventricular tachycardia or atrial fibrillation with bundle branch block?

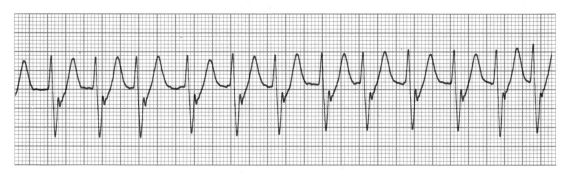

Because of the rapid rate, it is very easy to overlook the irregular ventricular rate and identify the rhythm as ventricular tachycardia. But because of the ventricular irregularity and the absence of P waves, the diagnosis of atrial fibrillation with bundle branch block is indicated.

Ventricular tachycardia or atrial fibrillation with bundle branch block?

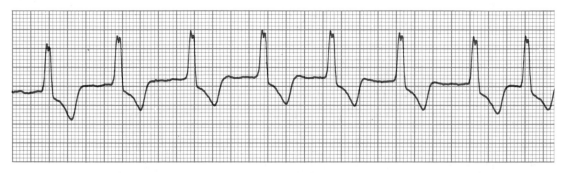

Initially, the ventricular rate appears regular, and with the widened QRS, ventricular tachycardia is suspected. But notice the subtle irregularity in the ventricular cycle, which leads one to suspect atrial fibrillation with bundle branch block.

Ventricular tachycardia or atrial fibrillation with bundle branch block?

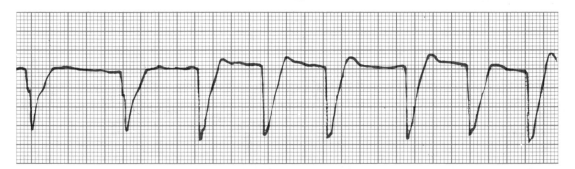

The wide and bizarre QRS complexes lead the casual observer to diagnose ventricular tachycardia immediately. However, the very irregular ventricular rate is the clue to the correct diagnosis: atrial fibrillation with bundle branch block.

Ventricular tachycardia or junctional tachycardia with bundle branch block?

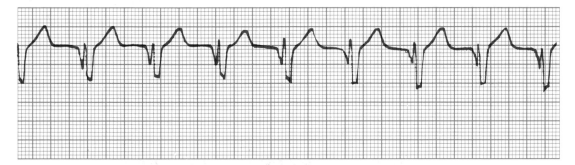

This strip demonstrates no P waves and a ventricular rate that is regular. QRS complexes are wide and bizarre. A diagnosis of accelerated idioventricular rhythm would be correct. But because of the absence of P waves and the regularity of rhythm, this could also be correctly identified as a junctional tachycardia with bundle branch block. A good guideline to follow is that if there is no record of bundle branch block in the patient's history, it is better to avoid the use of the term.

Artifact or ventricular fibrillation?

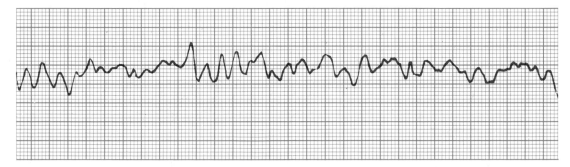

An ECG recorded with loose electrodes *can* produce this type of ECG strip. But this particular strip actually indicates ventricular fibrillation in a patient who soon died. If the patient from whom such a tracing is made is alert and responsive, one can assume that artifact has caused the erratic recording. Check the electrode connections on the patient and at the monitoring machine and begin recording again.

VENTRICULAR ECTOPIC RHYTHMS

Ventricular tachycardia or rate-related bundle branch block?

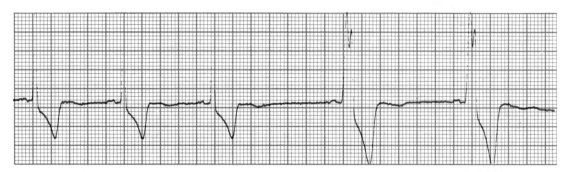

The P wave configuration and the PR interval remain constant throughout the strip. The QRS intermittently widens to greater than .11 second, demonstrating rate-related bundle branch block as the sinus cycle shows. Ventricular tachycardia is ruled out because of the sinus P wave preceding each widened QRS with a constant PR interval, signifying normal conduction.

Ventricular tachycardia or junctional tachycardia with bundle branch block?

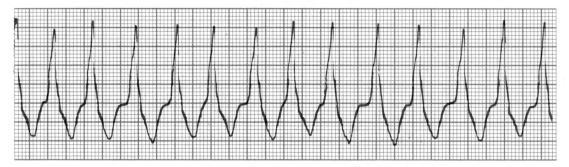

This rhythm is regular, has wide and bizarre QRS complexes, and shows no ectopic P waves. There is no evidence to suggest anything other than ventricular tachycardia.

Sinus tachycardia with bundle branch block or ventricular tachycardia?

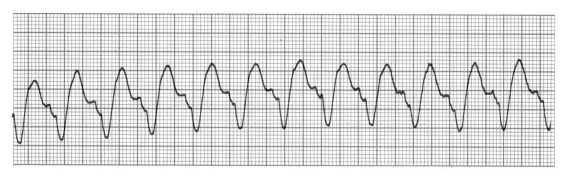

The presence of sinus P waves preceding each widened QRS complex cinches the diagnosis of sinus tachycardia with bundle branch block. Always check for sinus or ectopic P waves preceding each QRS with a constant PR interval before you make the diagnosis of ventricular tachycardia.

PRACTICE ECG STRIPS

I have purposely included artifact in some of the ECG strips to simulate the types of strips you might expect to find in the field. Eyeball the PR and QRS intervals for normal or abnormal intervals rather than exact measurements. Estimate the rate, identify the rhythm, and label any arrhythmias present.

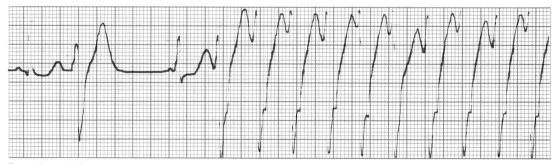

Practice strip 1

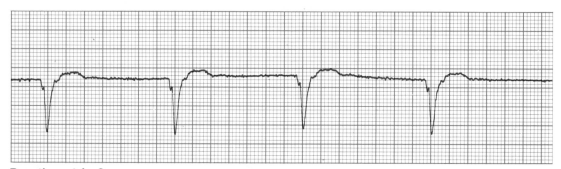

Practice strip 2

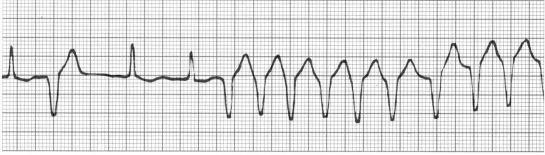

Practice strip 3

HOW TO QUICKLY AND ACCURATELY MASTER ARRHYTHMIA INTERPRETATION

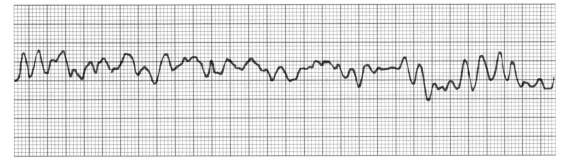

Practice strip 4

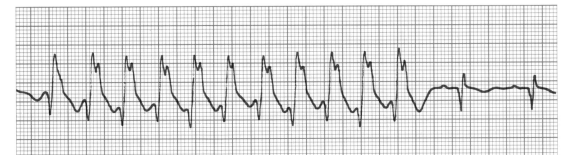

Practice strip 5

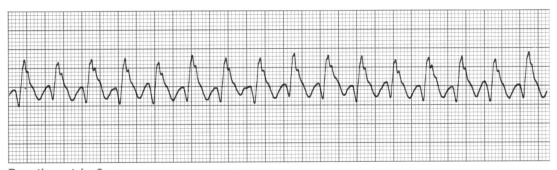

Practice strip 6

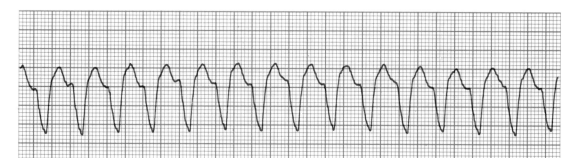

Practice strip 7

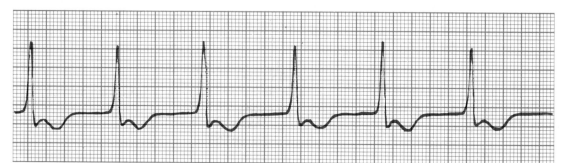

Practice strip 8

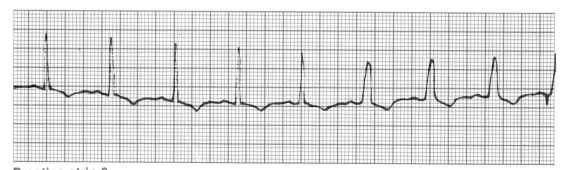

Practice strip 9

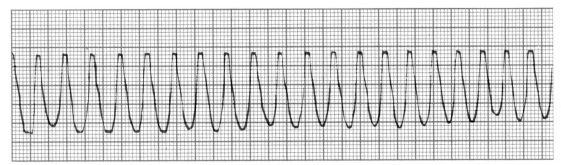

Practice strip 10

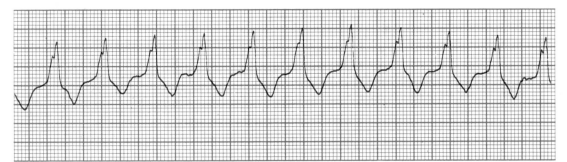

Practice strip 11

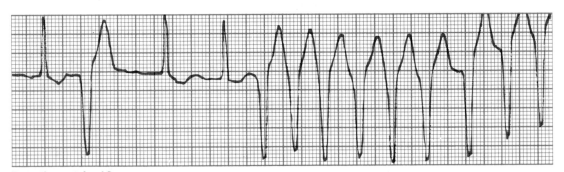

Practice strip 12

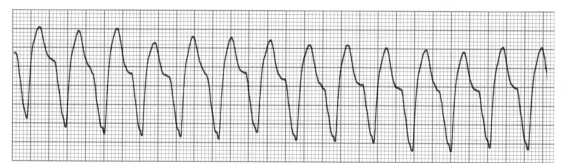

Practice strip 13

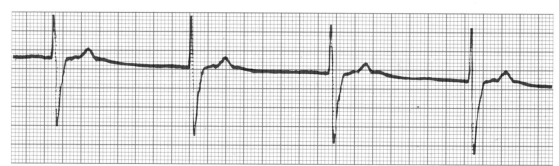

Practice strip 14

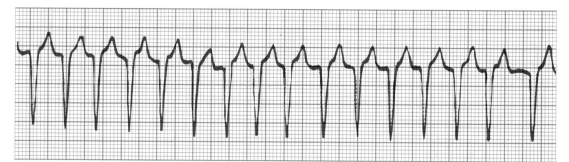

Practice strip 15

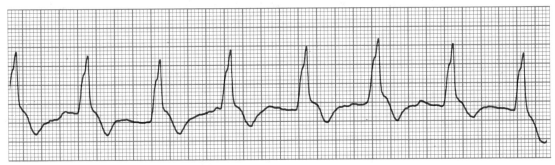

Practice strip 16

PRACTICE ECG STRIP ANSWERS

1. Sinus rhythm with an isolated VPC and a run of ventricular tachycardia initiated by a fusion beat

2. Accelerated idioventricular rhythm

3. Atrial fibrillation with an isolated VPC and a run of ventricular tachycardia initiated by a malignant VPC

4. Ventricular fibrillation

5. Ventricular tachycardia and conversion to sinus rhythm

6. Ventricular tachycardia

7. Ventricular tachycardia

8. Accelerated idioventricular rhythm

9. Sinus rhythm and intermittent bundle branch block

10. Ventricular flutter

11. Ventricular tachycardia

12. Atrial fibrillation with one isolated VPC and a run of ventricular tachycardia

13. Ventricular tachycardia

14. Probable junctional escape rhythm with bundle branch block. Notice the inverted ectopic P waves buried in each T wave

15. Atrial fibrillation

16. Accelerated idioventricular rhythm with some visible sinus P waves demonstrating AV dissociation

Chapter 9

ABERRATION AND WOLFF–PARKINSON–WHITE SYNDROME

ABERRATION

Aberration is a temporary variation or change in the QRS complex from the normal configuration, and it occurs when a sinus or supraventricular impulse activates the ventricles in an abnormal way. An impulse travels down the conduction pathways and finds one of the bundle branches to be refractory or busy from the previous beat, so conduction takes place abnormally from one ventricle to the other, through ventricular myocardium. Because of the delay in conduction, a wide and bizarre QRS complex results.

Aberration occurs if:

APCs or JPCs occur so close to the previous beat that one of the bundle branches is still refractory from the previous beat and cannot conduct the impulse

During irregular ventricular rates found in atrial fibrillation and atrial flutter, a long R-R cycle (when the refractory period of the bundle branches normally lengthens) is followed by a short R-R cycle and one of the bundle branches is still refractory and cannot conduct the impulse

Aberration can be an isolated event involving one or two beats, or it can occur for a longer period during tachycardia.

Aberration mimics VPCs and ventricular tachycardias. One must be able to differentiate between a supraventricular tachycardia with aberration and a true, life-threatening ventricular tachycardia. The rapid rates make distinctions difficult. Look for the clues of ectopic P waves buried in the T waves of the previous beats, or, in atrial fibrillation or atrial flutter, look for a long R-R cycle followed by a short R-R cycle.

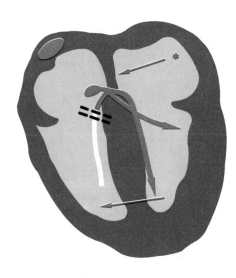

The following simplified criteria are used for recognition of aberration:

1. An APC with aberration is recognized by an early ectopic P wave preceding a wide and bizarre QRS.

2. A JPC with aberration is recognized by an inverted, early, ectopic P wave either preceding or immediately following a wide and bizarre QRS.

3. Atrial fibrillation or flutter with aberration is recognized by a long R-R cycle followed by a short R-R cycle, followed in turn by a wide and bizarre QRS.

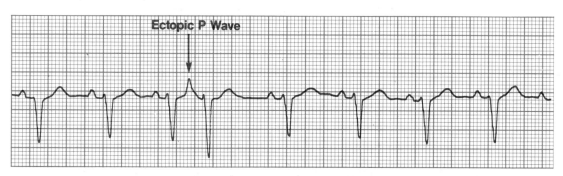

Sinus rhythm with bundle branch block and one APC with aberrancy. The ectopic P wave atop the preceding T wave is so obvious that there is no possibility of mislabeling this as a VPC.

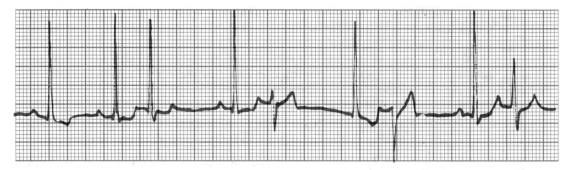

Sinus rhythm with four isolated APCs showing varying degrees of aberrancy. The second APC is followed by a junctional escape beat. Because the APCs arrive so early, they find one of the bundle branches busy from the previous beat. Aberrant beats are recorded because of the delay in conduction through abnormal conduction pathways. If the APCs arrive too early in the cycle, they may be nonconducted rather than displaying aberrancy.

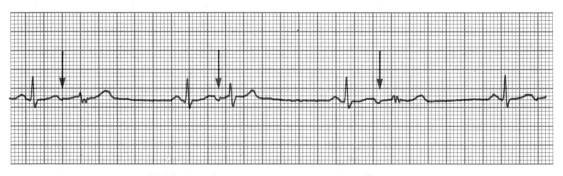

JPCs with aberrant conduction in bigeminy. These early ectopic beats should not be confused with VPCs because of the inverted ectopic P wave (*arrows*) preceding each one. These confirm the diagnosis of JPCs. Each JPC demonstrates varying degrees of aberrancy, depending on the prematurity of its arrival.

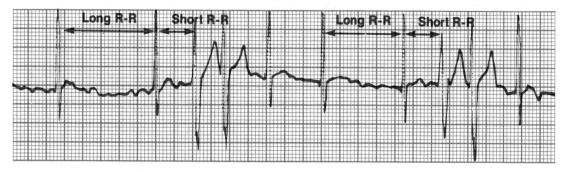

Atrial fibrillation with four beats displaying aberrancy. The long R-R cycle, followed closely by a short R-R cycle, favors the diagnosis of aberrancy.

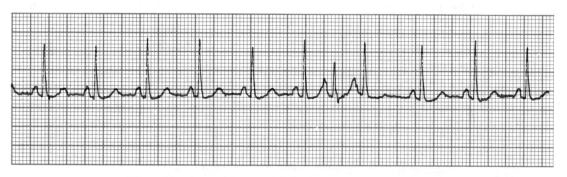

Sinus rhythm with two APCs in a row, the first displaying aberrancy. The ectopic P waves are seen atop the preceding T waves.

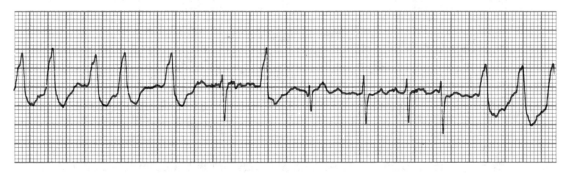

Atrial fibrillation with runs of aberrant beats. The runs of wide and bizarre beats demonstrate the same irregular ventricular response as does atrial fibrillation and rule out the diagnosis of ventricular tachycardia.

ABERRATION AND WOLFF–PARKINSON–WHITE SYNDROME

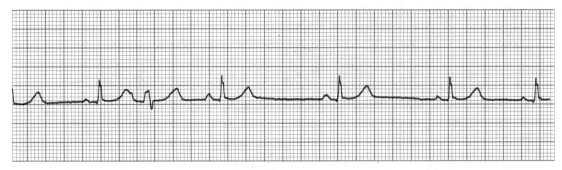

Sinus bradycardia with an APC with aberrancy. Note the early ectopic P wave deforming the T wave of the previous beat, ruling out the diagnosis of VPC.

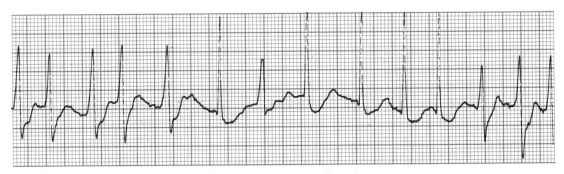

Atrial fibrillation with a run of aberrant beats, which display the characteristic irregular ventricular response of atrial fibrillation

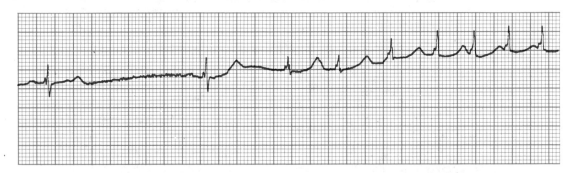

Sinus bradycardia with a run of supraventricular tachycardia with aberrancy. The QRS complex has not widened but has only altered its configuration slightly. The tachycardia starts out slowly and irregularly and then seems to regulate its rate as it continues, making it difficult to identify the exact supraventricular rhythm.

HOW TO QUICKLY AND ACCURATELY MASTER ARRHYTHMIA INTERPRETATION

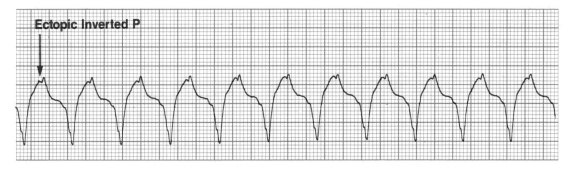

Junctional tachycardia with aberrancy. Notice the ectopic inverted
P waves following each beat atop the T waves, confirming the
diagnosis of junctional tachycardia. The beats display aberrancy
because of the rapid rate.

WOLFF–PARKINSON–WHITE SYNDROME

In Wolff–Parkinson–White syndrome (WPW) an accessory conduction pathway is present between the atria and the ventricles. This pathway allows impulses to be conducted to the ventricles faster than by way of the AV node. WPW is characterized by a shortened PR interval, as the impulse conducts rapidly to the ventricles via an accessary pathway; a slurring of the initial portion of the QRS (the *delta wave*), as one ventricle is depolarized rapidly through an abnormal conduction pathway and the other often through the normal pathway; and often a widened QRS complex, when both ventricles are depolarized solely by conduction through the accessory pathway. There are varying degrees of slurring and widening, depending on the contribution of each conduction pathway to ventricular activation.

DELTA WAVES

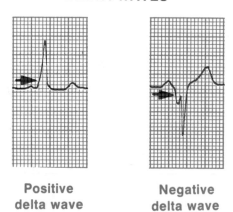

Positive
delta wave

Negative
delta wave

WPW is associated with supraventricular tachycardias that tend to mimic ventricular tachycardia because of the widened QRS complex. Differentiation between supraventricular tachycardia with aberration (because of the longer period of refractivity of one of the bundle branches) and supraventricular tachycardia with WPW (because of an accessory pathway to the ventricles) can be impossible in rapid tracings. Just the knowledge that a supraventricular tachycardia is occurring rather than a ventricular tachycardia is sufficient information during emergency monitoring.

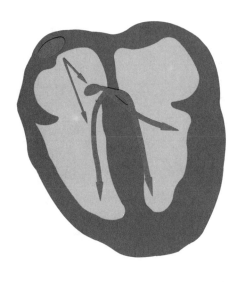

The following criteria are used for recognition of WPW:

1. In sinus rhythm, the PR interval is short because of conduction through an accessory pathway to the ventricles.
2. A delta wave is present.
3. There is a variation in the widening of the QRS complex.
4. Intermittent episodes of supraventricular tachycardia occur with widened QRS complexes and delta waves.

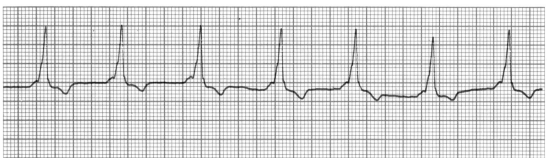

WPW displaying the shortened PR interval and delta wave. The PR is short but constant, ruling out AV dissociation. The shortened PR and the delta wave differentiate this from bundle branch block.

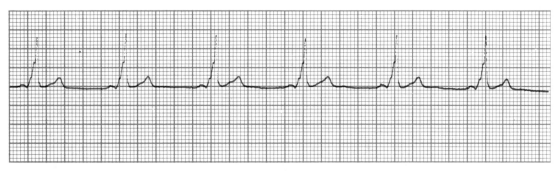

WPW displaying the characteristic shortened PR interval and a delta wave.

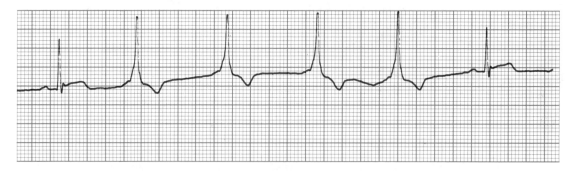

Sinus rhythm with normal PR and QRS intervals and intermittent WPW, displaying shortened PR intervals and widened QRS complexes for four beats and then a return to normal conduction.

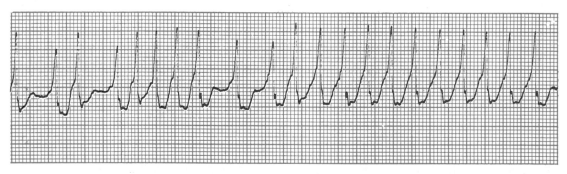

Atrial fibrillation is present, as noted by the irregular ventricular response. The QRS is widened, which leads one to diagnose bundle branch block, but the delta wave that is present confirms the diagnosis of atrial fibrillation with WPW.

DIFFERENTIAL DIAGNOSIS

VPC or supraventricular premature beat with aberrancy?

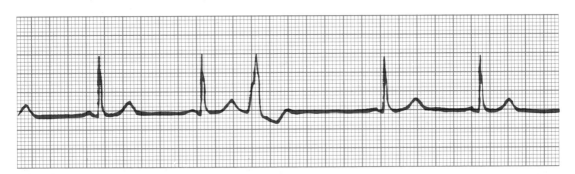

The premature beat is wide and bizarre, and there is no evidence of an ectopic P wave. The interpretation is sinus bradycardia with one isolated VPC.

VPCs and APCs or all APCs?

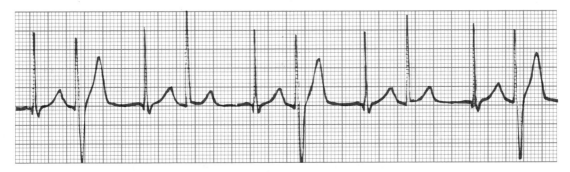

Every other beat is premature. Every other premature beat meets the criteria for APC because the T waves of the previous beats are distorted with an ectopic P wave. The questionable premature beats have the same distortion in the preceding T waves and therefore fit the criteria for APCs with aberrancy. This strip represents APCs in bigeminy with alternate APCs displaying aberrancy.

Is the labeled beat (*arrow*) an APC with aberrancy or a fusion beat?

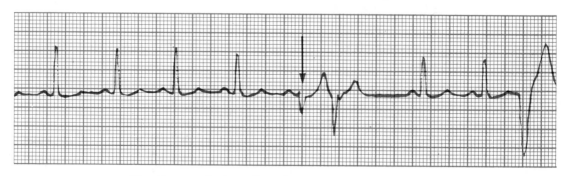

The P wave before the wide and bizarre QRS is not premature and
therefore not an APC. The P wave is a sinus P wave and is followed
by a pair of VPCs, the first a fusion beat. An additional isolated VPC
is seen.

Atrial flutter with two isolated VPCs or aberrant beats?

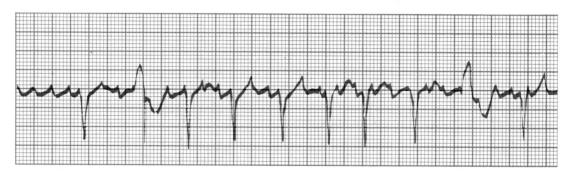

The two questionable beats recorded with the atrial flutter with
variable block do not come sufficiently early in the cycle to warrant
use of the term *aberrancy*. The two beats are probably unifocal
VPCs.

Atrial fibrillation with three aberrant beats or three VPCs?

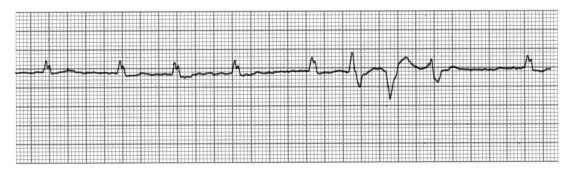

Aberration will not usually demonstrate alternate shifts in direction at this rate. These beats represent three multifocal VPCs in a row during atrial fibrillation.

Sinus rhythm with run of ventricular tachycardia or atrial tachycardia with aberrancy?

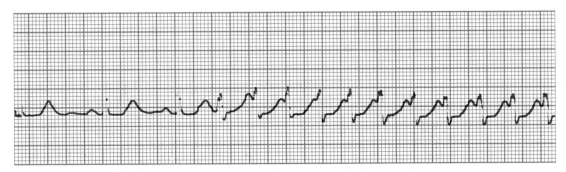

The first beat of the tachycardia displays an ectopic P wave in the T wave of the previous beat, giving credence to the diagnosis of atrial tachycardia with aberrancy.

ABERRATION AND WOLFF–PARKINSON–WHITE SYNDROME

PRACTICE ECG STRIPS

I have purposely included artifact in some of the ECG strips to simulate the types of strips you might expect to find in the field. Eyeball the PR and QRS intervals for normal or abnormal intervals rather than exact measurements. Estimate the rate, identify the rhythm, and label any arrhythmias present.

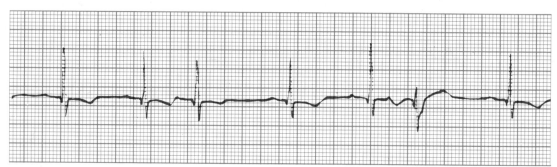

Practice strip 1

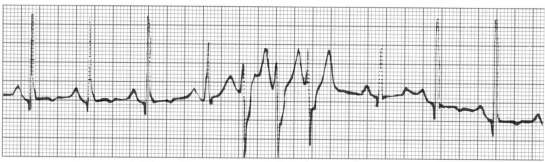

Practice strip 2

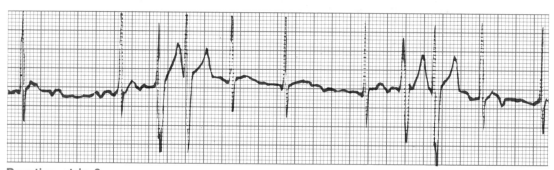

Practice strip 3

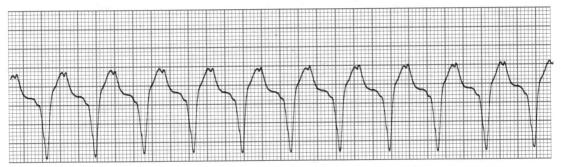

Practice strip 4

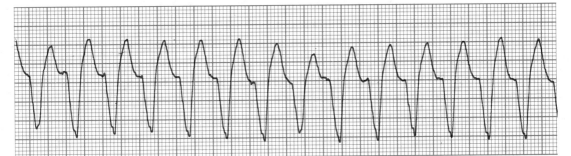

Practice strip 5

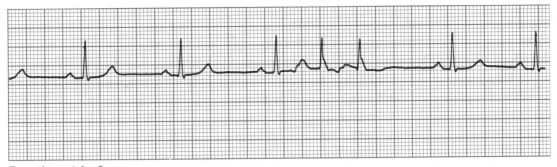

Practice strip 6

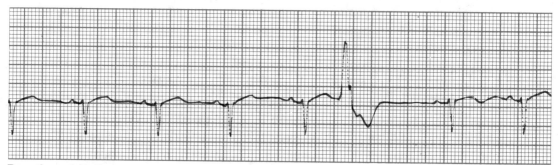

Practice strip 7

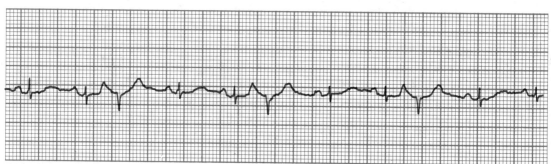

Practice strip 8

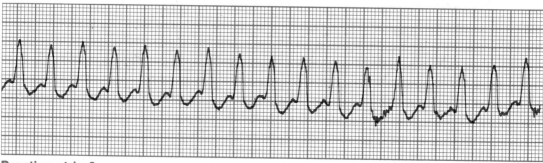

Practice strip 9

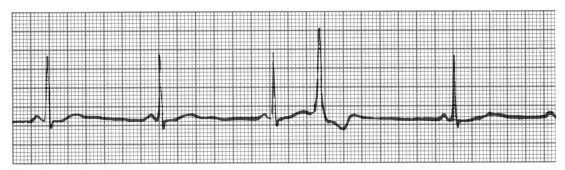

Practice strip 10

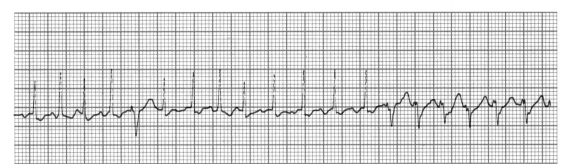

Practice strip 11

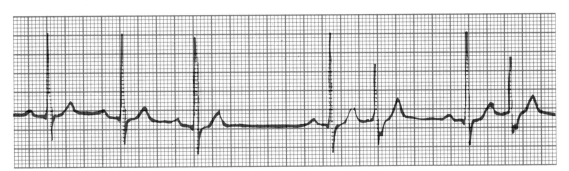

Practice strip 12

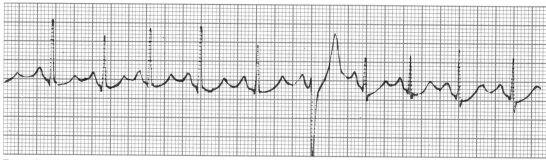

Practice strip 13

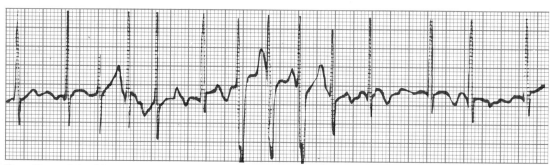

Practice strip 14

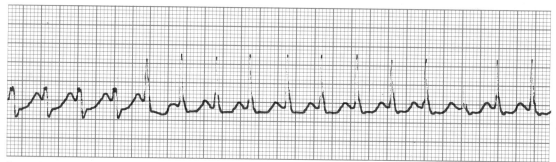

Practice strip 15

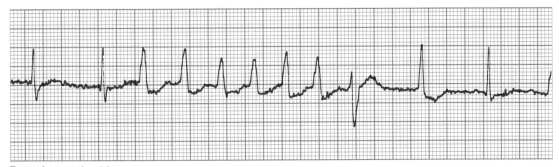

Practice strip 16

PRACTICE ECG STRIP ANSWERS

1. Sinus rhythm with two isolated APCs, the second displaying aberration
2. Sinus rhythm with four unifocal VPCs in a row, the first of them a fusion beat
3. Atrial fibrillation with four aberrant beats
4. Junctional tachycardia with aberrancy
5. Ventricular tachycardia
6. Sinus bradycardia with a pair of APCs with aberrancy
7. Sinus rhythm with one isolated VPC
8. Sinus rhythm with APCs with aberrancy in trigeminy
9. Ventricular tachycardia
10. Sinus bradycardia with one isolated VPC
11. Atrial fibrillation with aberration
12. Sinus rhythm with APCs in bigeminy, the first nonconducted and the other two with aberration
13. Sinus tachycardia with one end diastolic VPC
14. Atrial fibrillation with aberrant beats
15. Atrial tachycardia with aberration, reverting to atrial tachycardia with normal conduction
16. Atrial fibrillation with aberrant beats and one VPC

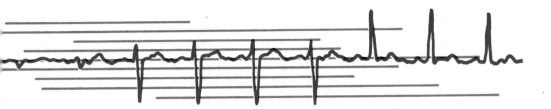

Chapter 10
AV BLOCK

The delay or blockage of sinus or other supraventricular impulses through the AV node is called AV block. When we consider nonconducted APCs, atrial flutter with varying conduction, PAT with block, and aberration, we are referring to the physiological refractivity of the conduction system; it is impossible for the heart to conduct normally when it has not yet recovered from another impulse. This is considered normal and prevents the heart from contracting too rapidly; however, when an impulse *should* be conducted and is not, it is considered AV block.

When the heart is in sinus rhythm and AV block is present, the P-P cycle is regular, but each P wave is not always followed by a QRS complex. These isolated P waves are called *dropped P waves*. AV block exhibits ventricular pauses and/or slow ventricular rates.

FIRST DEGREE AV BLOCK

First degree AV block has been demonstrated in previous chapters and is characterized by a PR interval greater than .20 second due to the prolongation of the refractory period in the AV node. This arrhythmia is common and not dangerous.

SECOND DEGREE AV BLOCK
WENCKEBACH

In second degree AV block Wenckebach, the conduction of sinus or other supraventricular impulses to the ventricles becomes increasingly more difficult, causing progressively longer PR intervals until a P wave is not conducted. The pause following the dropped P wave enables the AV node to recover, and the following P wave is conducted with a normal or slightly shorter PR interval. The R-R intervals in each sequence become progressively shorter until the pause occurs. A junctional or ventricular escape beat may terminate the pause. This arrhythmia is not considered dangerous or life threatening and does not progress to a more serious AV block.

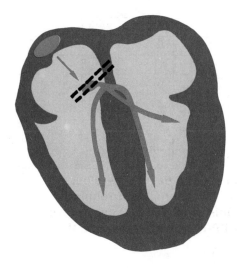

The following simplified criteria are used for recognition of second degree AV block Wenckebach:

1. The PR progressively lengthens from beat to beat until a sinus P wave is not conducted and a ventricular pause occurs.
2. The P-P intervals are constant.

When you view an entire ECG strip, you will see a ventricular pattern emerge with this arrhythmia. On the first strip below there appear to be QRS complexes grouped as pairs. This is due to the Wenckebach sequence of a normal P wave with first degree AV block as the first beat of the sequence, the prolonged PR as the second beat, and the dropped P wave as the third beat with no QRS following it. This leaves a pair of QRS complexes for each Wenckebach sequence. This type of pattern is called second degree AV block Wenckeback with a 3:2 sequence—there are three P waves and only two QRS complexes in each sequence.

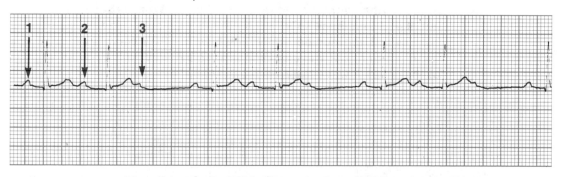

The strip begins with sinus rhythm with first degree AV block, then there is a PR interval that becomes longer by the second beat and an isolated sinus P wave with no QRS (dropped P wave) as the third beat in the sequence. The P-P cycle is regular—the dropped P wave occurs exactly on time, so it is not an early nonconducted APC but second degree AV block Wenckebach. The cycle then repeats. There are three P waves for two QRS complexes in each cycle, making this a 3:2 Wenckebach sequence.

AV BLOCK

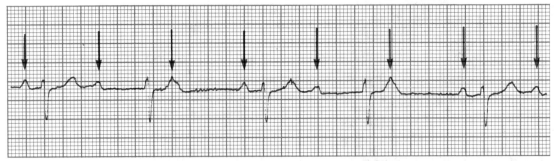

Sinus rhythm with first degree and second degree AV block Wenckebach with a 3:2 sequence. The ventricular irregularity of Wenckebach is not so obvious in this strip. The P-P cycle (*arrows*) is regular. Notice how the dropped P waves are hidden in the T waves.

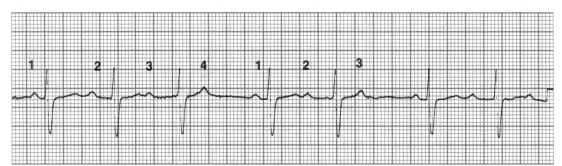

Sinus rhythm with second degree AV block Wenckebach with an initial 4:3 sequence followed by a 3:2 sequence. The P waves of both cycles are numbered. Notice how the PR intervals gradually lengthen until a P wave is dropped. The P-P cycle is regular—none of the sinus P waves are early.

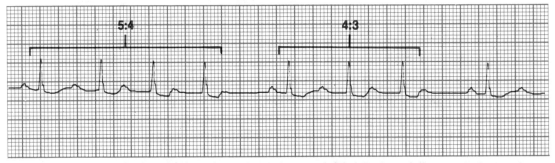

Sinus rhythm demonstrating an initial 5:4 and then a 4:3 sequence in second degree AV block Wenckebach. The PR lengthening in each cycle is evident.

HOW TO QUICKLY AND ACCURATELY MASTER ARRHYTHMIA INTERPRETATION

SECOND DEGREE
AV BLOCK MOBITZ

In second degree AV block Mobitz the conduction of sinus or other supraventricular impulses to the ventricles occurs with intermittent block of some of the P waves. The PR interval is constant and does not lengthen before a dropped P wave as it does in second degree AV block Wenckebach. No more than one P wave in a row is nonconducted, and the ventricular pauses that occur are sometimes terminated by junctional or ventricular escape beats. This arrhythmia is considered dangerous and often progresses to more serious forms of AV block. The slow ventricular rates accompanying this arrhythmia may cause patient discomfort.

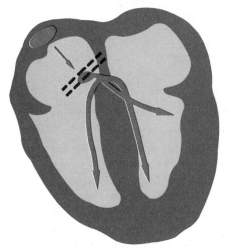

The following simplified criteria are used for recognition of second degree AV block Mobitz:

1. The PR interval is constant, the P-P cycle is regular, and a sinus P wave is dropped, producing a ventricular pause.
2. No more than one sinus P wave is dropped in a row.

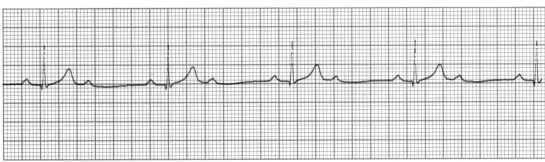

Sinus rhythm with first degree AV block with alternating P waves conducted to the ventricles, demonstrating second degree AV block Mobitz. The P-P cycle is regular, and only alternating P waves are conducted to the ventricles to produce a QRS complex. The PR interval remains constant.

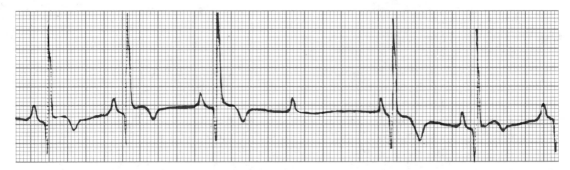

Sinus rhythm with one episode of second degree AV block Mobitz

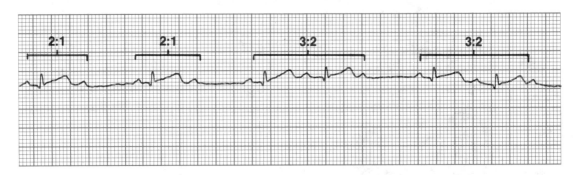

Sinus rhythm with what appears to be both second degree AV block Mobitz and Wenckebach in the same strip. The first and second sequences show constant PR intervals and dropped P waves, suggesting AV block Mobitz. The last two sequences show a progressive increase in the PR interval before a dropped P wave, confirming the diagnosis of AV block Wenckebach. The first two sequences also represent 2:1 Wenckebach, in which the PR interval has no opportunity to lengthen. Without the presence of a 3:2 sequence in the strip confirming the diagnosis of AV block Wenckebach, the diagnosis of AV block Mobitz should be presumed. During emergency monitoring it would be better to err on the side of safety, assume that AV block Mobitz is present, and treat it accordingly than to underestimate the severity of the problem.

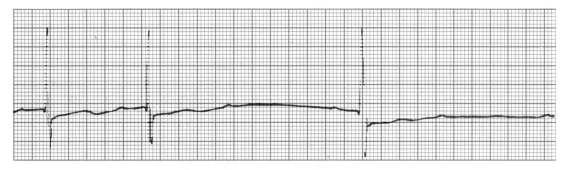

Sinus bradycardia with first degree AV block and second degree AV block Mobitz with a slow ventricular response of approximately 25 beats per minute. Without evidence of a Wenckebach sequence, demonstrated by a progressive lengthening of a PR interval before a dropped P wave, AV block Mobitz should always be assumed.

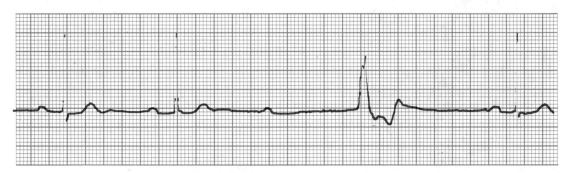

Sinus bradycardia with first degree and second degree AV block Mobitz. The ventricular pause caused by the AV block is terminated by a ventricular escape beat.

HIGH GRADE AV BLOCK

High grade AV block is the conduction of sinus or other supraventricular impulses to the ventricles with intermittent block of more than one P wave in a row. The ventricular rate can be very slow because of the blocked P waves, and these pauses may be terminated by junctional or ventricular escape beats. Atrial fibrillation and flutter with high grade AV block produce long ventricular pauses. This arrhythmia is considered very dangerous because of the slow heart rates and because it often progresses to complete AV block.

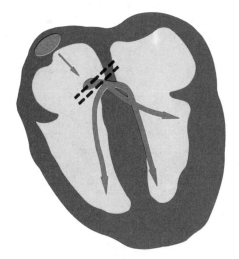

The following simplified criteria are used for recognition of high grade AV block:

1. The PR interval is constant, the P-P cycle is regular, and there are two or more dropped P waves for each QRS complex, producing a ventricular pause.

2. In sinus rhythm the PR interval is constant.

3. In atrial fibrillation or flutter, long ventricular pauses are present.

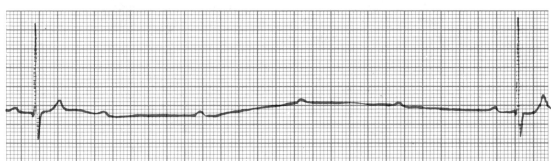

Sinus rhythm with first degree AV block and high grade AV block. The P-P cycle is regular, and the PR interval is constant when conduction occurs. There are four dropped P waves during the long ventricular pause, and no escape mechanism comes to the rescue. The fifth sinus P wave finally conducts to the ventricles, making this 5:1 high grade AV block. Five P waves are required to produce a QRS complex in this strip.

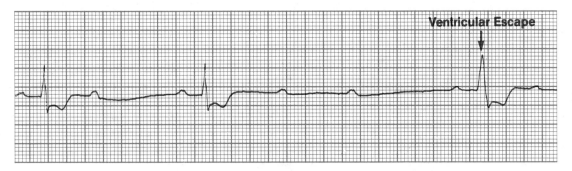

Sinus bradycardia with first degree and second degree AV block Mobitz alternating with high grade AV block. The pause following the high grade block is terminated by a ventricular escape beat.

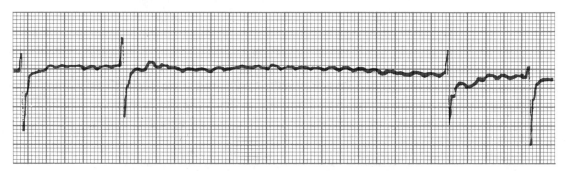

Atrial fibrillation with a long ventricular pause demonstrating high grade AV block

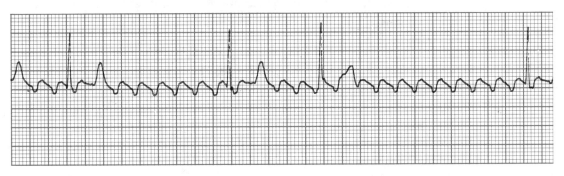

Atrial flutter with varying block and a slow ventricular rate with long ventricular pauses, depicting high grade AV block

AV BLOCK

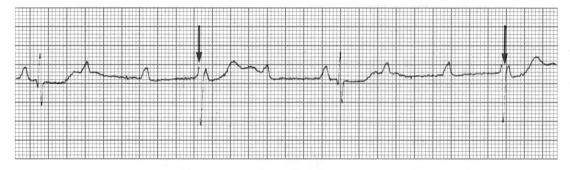

Sinus rhythm with high grade AV block and intermittent ventricular
escape beats (*arrows*) terminating the ventricular pauses

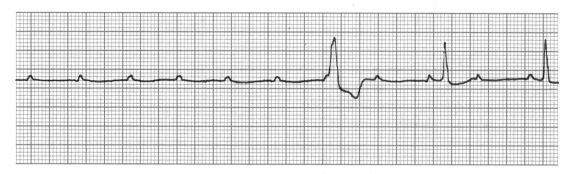

Sinus tachycardia with high grade AV block and a long ventricular
pause finally terminated by a ventricular escape beat. Although the
strip is not sufficiently long to demonstrate it, the ventricular pause
lasts 15 seconds. Second degree AV block Mobitz then commences
as the underlying heart rhythm.

COMPLETE AV BLOCK

In complete AV block there is no conduction between the atria and the ventricles, and the atria and ventricles beat independently under the control of separate pacemaking foci. In sinus rhythm the PR interval is constantly changing because the P waves and the QRS complexes bear no relationship to each other, and conduction between them does not occur. The atria are under the control of a sinus or supraventricular pacemaker, and the ventricles are rescued by either a junctional or a ventricular escape rhythm.

Although this arrhythmia appears very similar to AV dissociation, complete AV block is a permanent lack of conduction between the atria and ventricles. The ventricular rates are slow because an escape mechanism rescues the heart. In AV dissociation the lack of conduction between the atria and ventricles is temporary, and the atrial and ventricular rates are often similar, whereas the ventricular rates are substantially slower than the atrial rates in complete AV block.

Atrial fibrillation normally produces an extremely irregular ventricular response. But in the presence of complete AV block, when none of the fibrillatory waves are conducted to the ventricles, an escape rhythm takes control of pacing the ventricles, and the ventricular response becomes uncharacteristically regular.

Complete AV block is a very serious arrhythmia because the ventricular rates are often too slow to maintain adequate systemic circulation and because ventricular standstill and death will occur if an escape mechanism does not function and a pacemaker is not inserted.

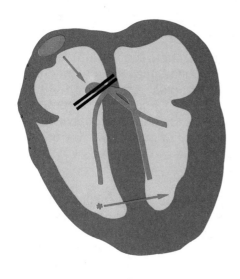

The following simplified criteria are used for recognition of complete AV block:

1. There is a permanent lack of conduction between the atria and ventricles.

2. The atria are under the control of a sinus or supraventricular focus, and the ventricles are controlled by either a junctional or a ventricular escape rhythm. The atrial and ventricular rates are usually regular, but not at the same rate. The ventricular rate is usually considerably slower than the atrial rate.

3. In sinus rhythm the PR varies because the P wave bears no relationship to the QRS.

4. In atrial fibrillation the ventricular rate is slow and regular because a junctional or ventricular escape rhythm takes control of the ventricles.

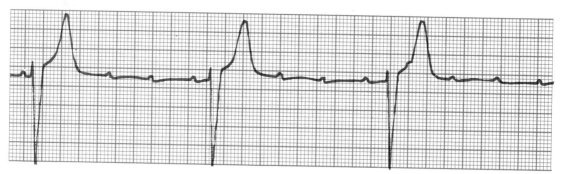

Sinus tachycardia with complete heart block and a ventricular escape rhythm. The P-P and R-R cycles are regular but at different rates, and the PR interval varies, confirming the permanent absence of conduction between the atria and ventricles. The slow ventricular rate and the widened QRS confirm the presence of a ventricular escape rhythm.

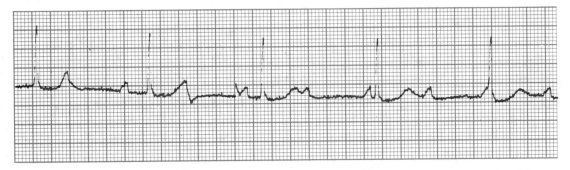

Both the atrial and ventricular rates are regular—but each at completely different rates. The PR interval constantly varies, confirming the lack of conduction between the atria and ventricles and establishing the diagnosis of complete AV block. Sinus rhythm is present in the atria, and the ventricles are controlled by an escape rhythm originating in the AV node. As you have learned previously, if the QRS is wide and bizarre, the escape rhythm originates in the ventricles; if the QRS complex is less than .11 second, the escape rhythm is junctional.

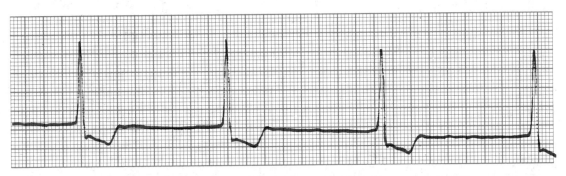

The baseline shows fine atrial fibrillatory waves, but the ventricular response is regular, which is uncharacteristic of atrial fibrillation. Because of the slowness and regularity of the ventricular response, complete AV block with a ventricular escape rhythm controlling the ventricles is suspected.

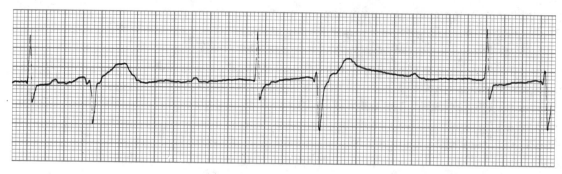

Sinus rhythm with complete AV block and a junctional escape rhythm with unifocal VPCs in bigeminy

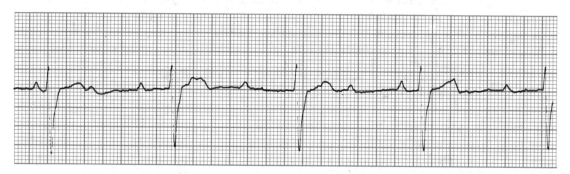

Sinus rhythm with complete AV block and a ventricular escape rhythm. The atrial and ventricular rates are regular but at different rates, and the PR interval varies, validating the diagnosis.

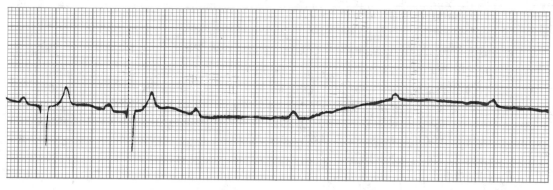

Sinus bradycardia with first degree AV block followed by complete AV block with ventricular standstill. An escape mechanism rescued the heart after 11 seconds.

DIFFERENTIAL DIAGNOSIS

AV block Wenckebach or nonconducted APCs?

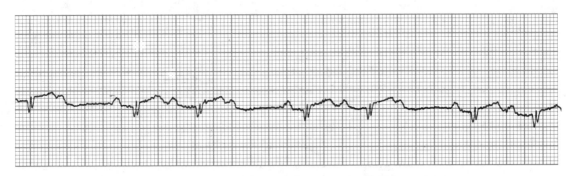

Check the P-P cycle and notice its regularity. None of the P waves are early, ruling out APCs, which are always premature. The PR interval becomes progressively longer until a P wave is dropped. This is sinus rhythm with first degree AV block and second degree AV block Wenckebach.

AV block Wenckebach or nonconducted APC?

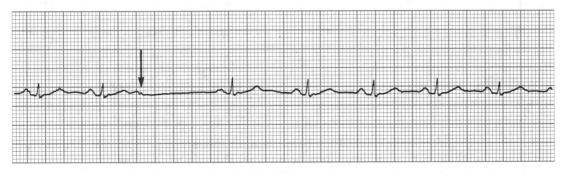

All the P waves are on time except the one buried in the T wave (*arrow*). Because it is early and its configuration differs from that of the sinus P waves, it represents an ectopic P wave or a nonconducted APC followed by an expected pause.

Sinus bradycardia with nonconducted APCs in bigeminy or AV block Mobitz?

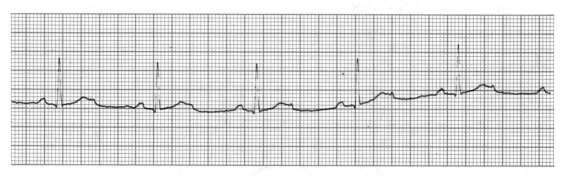

On inspection, there are P waves buried in all the T waves. When you "eyeball" the P-P cycle, all the P waves arrive at a regular interval, ruling out APCs, which are always premature. This is second degree AV block Mobitz.

AV block Wenckebach with 2:1 sequences or AV block Mobitz?

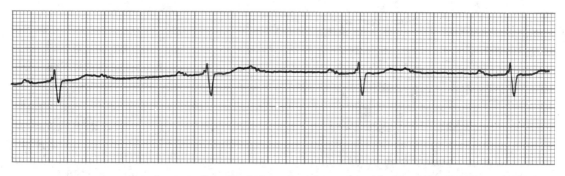

It is impossible to determine from this short strip which type of AV block is present. Unless another Wenckebach sequence that can show the PR interval lengthening occurs, second degree AV block Mobitz should be assumed.

Fine atrial fibrillation with complete AV block and a junctional escape rhythm or simply a junctional escape rhythm?

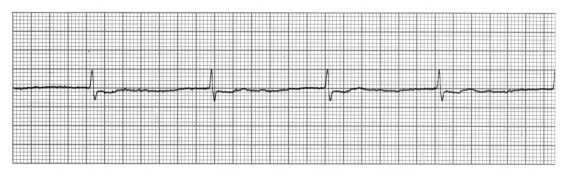

Unless ectopic P waves or atrial fibrillatory waves are visible, there is no way to differentiate between these two arrhythmias in a short strip. The better interpretation would simply be junctional escape rhythm unless you can verify atrial fibrillation from a history.

AV block Wenckebach or complete AV block?

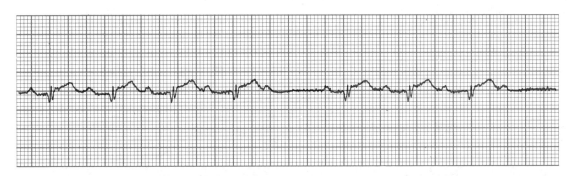

The PR intervals vary, the atrial and ventricular rates are different, and there is a progressive PR lengthening before each dropped P wave. The ventricular rate is not regular, as one would expect if complete AV block were present, and all the criteria point toward the interpretation of second degree AV block Wenckebach.

AV dissociation or complete AV block?

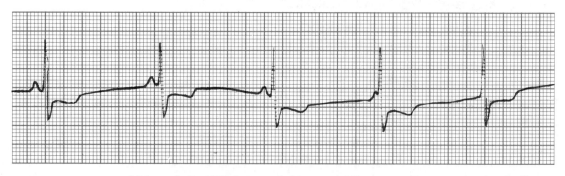

Although the PR intervals vary and there are two separate rhythms occurring, this is not complete AV block. The two heart rates are almost identical, which normally does not occur in complete AV block, and the P wave floats into the QRS complexes, giving credence to the diagnosis of AV dissociation. Complete AV block would normally have a ventricular rate much lower than the atrial rate.

PRACTICE ECG STRIPS

I have purposely included artifact in some of the ECG strips to simulate the types of strips you might expect to find in the field. Eyeball the PR and QRS intervals for normal or abnormal intervals rather than exact measurements. Estimate the rate, identify the rhythm, and label any arrhythmias present.

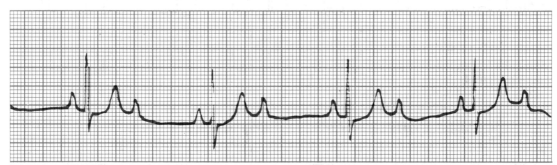

Practice strip 1

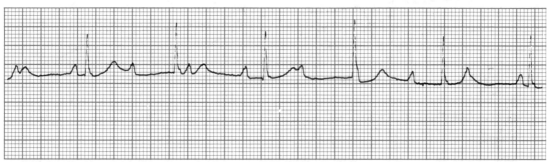

Practice strip 2

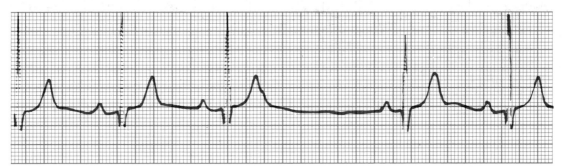

Practice strip 3

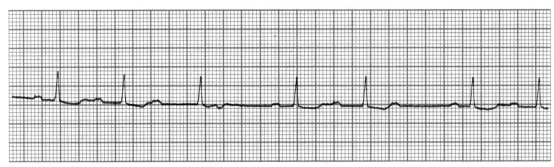

Practice strip 4

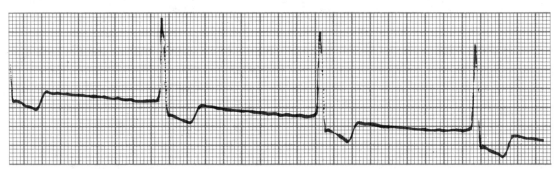

Practice strip 5

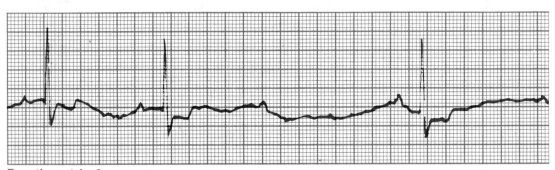

Practice strip 6

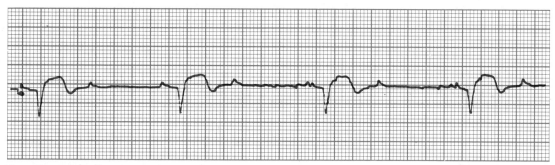

Practice strip 7

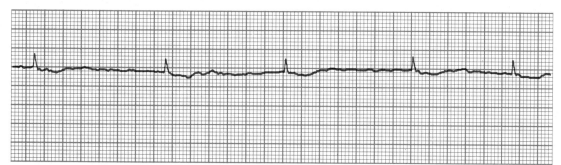

Practice strip 8

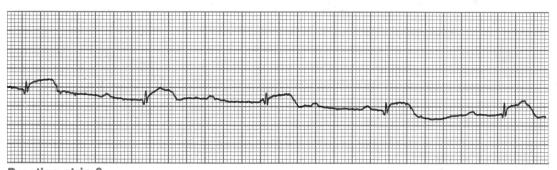

Practice strip 9

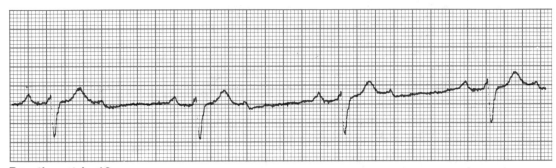

Practice strip 10

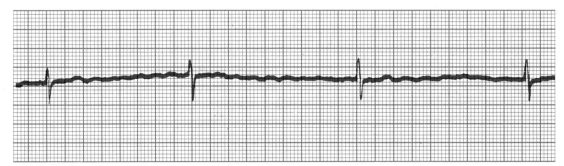

Practice strip 11

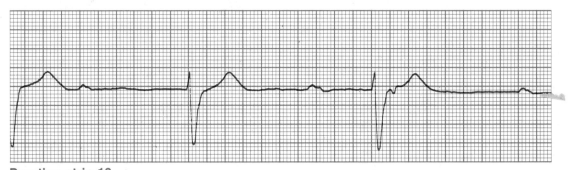

Practice strip 12

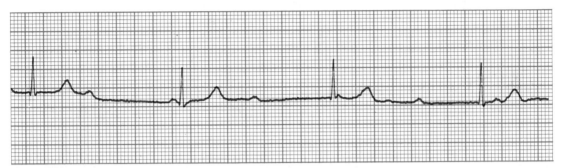

Practice strip 13

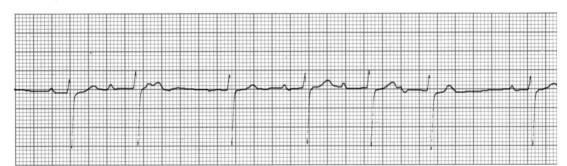

Practice strip 14

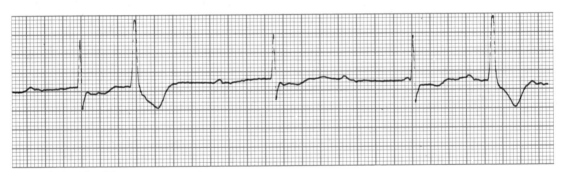

Practice strip 15

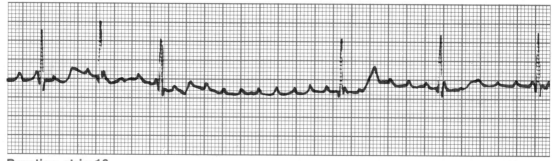

Practice strip 16

PRACTICE ECG STRIP ANSWERS

1. Sinus rhythm and second degree AV block Mobitz
2. Sinus rhythm, complete AV block, and a junctional escape rhythm
3. Sinus bradycardia with first degree AV block and a nonconducted APC
4. Sinus rhythm with first degree AV block and second degree AV block Wenckebach
5. Atrial fibrillation, complete AV block, and a ventricular escape rhythm
6. Sinus bradycardia and first and second degree AV block Mobitz
7. Sinus rhythm with second degree AV block Mobitz
8. Atrial fibrillation and high grade AV block
9. Sinus rhythm, complete AV block, and junctional escape rhythm
10. Sinus rhythm with a bundle branch block and first and second degree AV block Mobitz
11. Atrial fibrillation with high grade AV block
12. Sinus bradycardia and complete heart block with a ventricular escape rhythm
13. Sinus rhythm, complete AV block, and a junctional escape rhythm
14. Sinus rhythm with first and second degree AV block Wenckebach
15. Sinus rhythm with complete AV block, a junctional escape rhythm, and two unifocal VPCs
16. Atrial flutter with high grade AV block

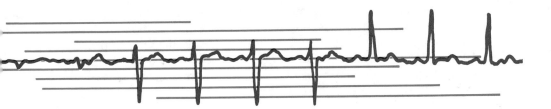

Chapter 11

SA BLOCK

SA block is a conduction disturbance between the sinus node and the surrounding atrial tissue that can cause delay or block in the conduction of sinus impulses to the atria. AV block, discussed in Chapter 10, is a delay or block in conduction in which P waves occur but QRS complexes are absent. In SA block the block or delay causes absence of both the P wave and the QRS complex.

FIRST DEGREE SA BLOCK

In first degree SA block all the sinus impulses are conducted to the atria, but with delay. This arrhythmia cannot be detected on an ECG strip.

SECOND DEGREE SA BLOCK

Second degree SA block is divided into two categories, similar to AV block. *Second degree SA block Wenckebach* is characterized by a ventricular pause that is preceded by progressively shorter P-P intervals and that measures less than twice the length of the preceding P-P interval.

Second degree SA block Mobitz is characterized by a P-P cycle of constant duration and a ventricular pause that measures two, three, or more times the length of the normal P-P interval. Junctional or ventricular escape beats may interrupt the ventricular pauses.

The following simplified criteria are used for recognition of second degree SA block Wenckebach:

1. The P-P cycles are progressively shorter before the pause.
2. The ventricular pause measures less than twice the length of the preceding P-P cycle.
3. The P wave and QRS complex are absent during the ventricular pause.

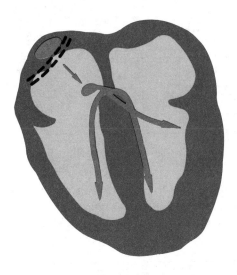

The following simplified criteria are used for recognition of second degree SA block Mobitz:

1. The P-P interval is constant.
2. The ventricular pause measures two, three, or more times the length of the normal P-P cycle.
3. The P waves and QRS complexes are absent during the ventricular pause.

Because differentiating between the two different types of SA block often requires careful measurements with calipers rather the eyeballing differences, the interpretation during monitoring out in the field and in emergencies should necessitate only the use of the category *SA block*. The general term *sinus arrest* is sometimes used instead. These arrhythmias usually do not cause serious emergencies because escape beats or rhythms usually terminate long pauses.

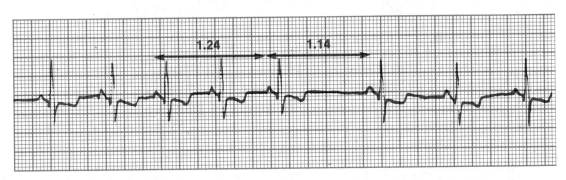

Sinus rhythm with the P-P interval becoming shorter before the pause and the pause measuring less than twice the preceding P-P interval. This demonstrates second degree SA block Wenckebach.

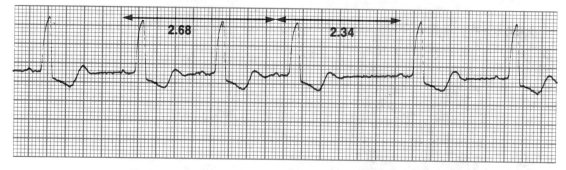

Sinus rhythm with bundle branch block. The P-P cycle shortens before the pause, and the pause measures less than twice the preceding P-P cycle. This represents second degree SA block Wenckebach.

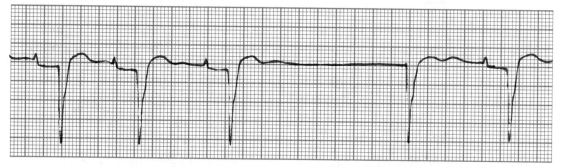

Sinus rhythm with first degree AV block and bundle branch block. The P-P cycle does not shorten before the pause, and the pause is terminated by a junctional escape beat. This strip demonstrates second degree SA block Mobitz.

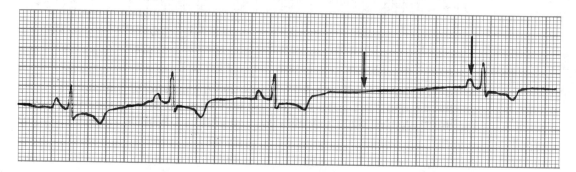

Sinus rhythm with one episode of 2:1 second degree SA block Mobitz. The P-P cycle remains constant before the pause, and the pause measures twice the preceding P-P interval. The sinus node has to fire twice before conduction to the atria occurs.

HOW TO QUICKLY AND ACCURATELY MASTER ARRHYTHMIA INTERPRETATION

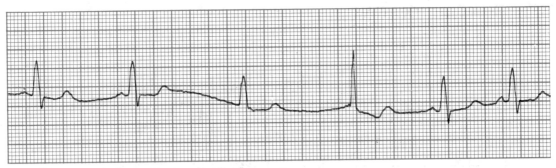

Sinus bradycardia with bundle branch block and an area of SA block terminated by two junctional escape beats and back to sinus rhythm

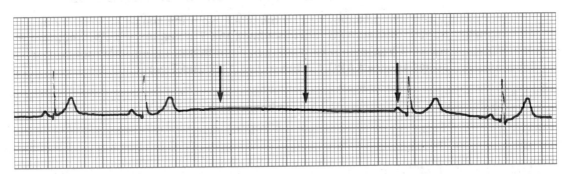

Sinus bradycardia with an episode of SA block Mobitz with 3 : 1 block. The sinus node has to fire three times before conduction to the atria is possible.

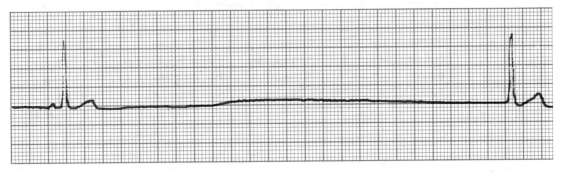

Sinus bradycardia with SA block and a junctional escape beat terminating the pause. The sinus P wave returned after 25 seconds. Because of the long ventricular pauses that continually occurred, a ventricular inhibited pacemaker was inserted.

SA BLOCK

DIFFERENTIAL DIAGNOSIS

SA block or nonconducted APC?

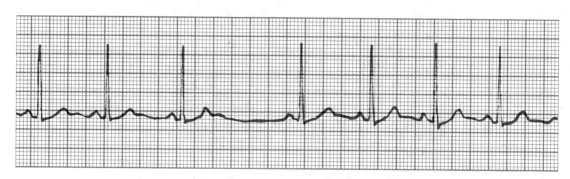

When trying to distinguish SA block from the pause caused by a nonconducted APC, always check the T wave for a hidden ectopic P wave. If you compare the T waves in this strip, you can notice the nonconducted APC hidden in the previous T wave.

SA block or nonconducted APC?

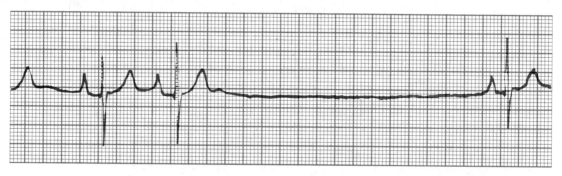

A nonconducted APC alone would never cause a long ventricular pause such as this. Without even checking the T wave, you can be certain that this is SA block.

SA block or sinus arrhythmia?

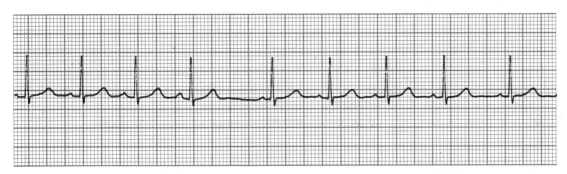

The ventricular pause is not particularly long in this strip, and there seems to be an ebb and flow to the rate because it is associated with respiration. This is sinus arrhythmia in a 24-year-old woman. Sinus arrhythmia is very common in children and young adults.

SA block or sinus arrhythmia?

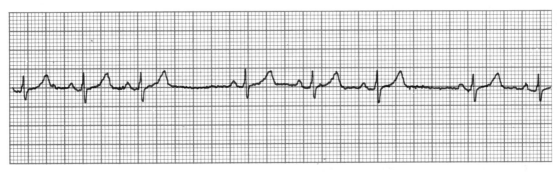

Although this strip meets all the criteria for second degree SA block Wenckebach, the facts that the patient is 8 years old and that there is evidence of respiratory variation in the heart rhythm give credence to the diagnosis of sinus arrhythmia.

SA block or sinus arrhythmia?

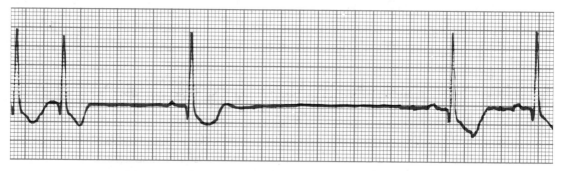

Sinus rhythm with one APC and an episode of 3:1 SA block. Sinus
arrhythmia would usually not cause such long ventricular pauses.

PRACTICE ECG STRIPS

I have purposely included artifact in some of the ECG strips to simulate the types of strips you might expect to find in the field. Eyeball
the PR and QRS intervals for normal or abnormal intervals rather
than exact measurements. Estimate the rate, identify the rhythm, and
label any arrhythmias present.

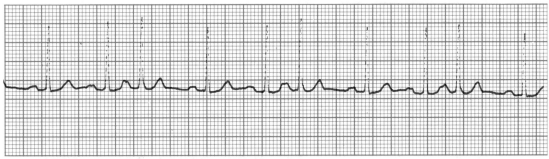

Practice strip 1

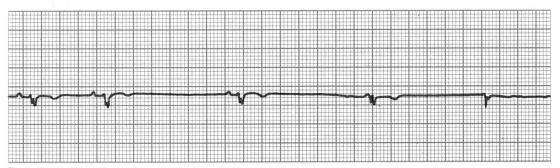

Practice strip 2

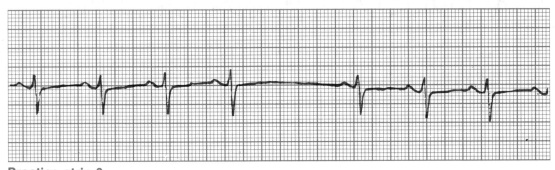

Practice strip 3

SA BLOCK

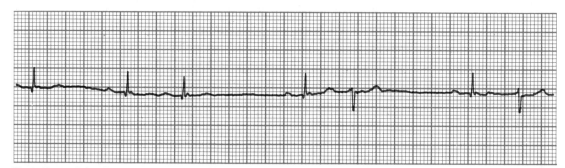

Practice strip 4

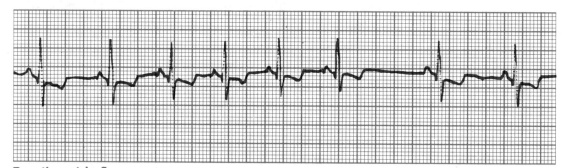

Practice strip 5

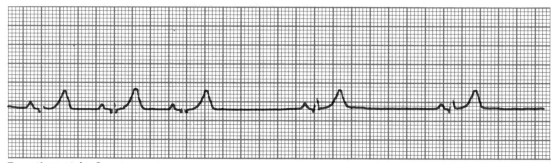

Practice strip 6

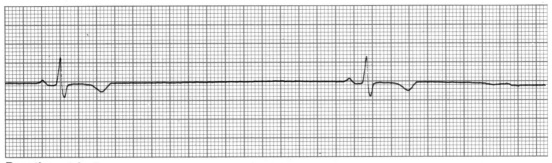

Practice strip 7

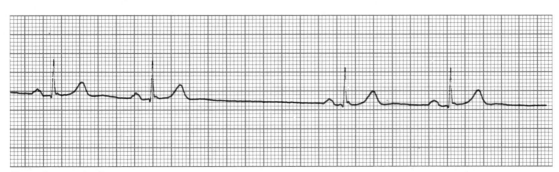

Practice strip 8

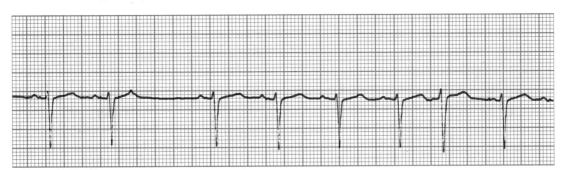

Practice strip 9

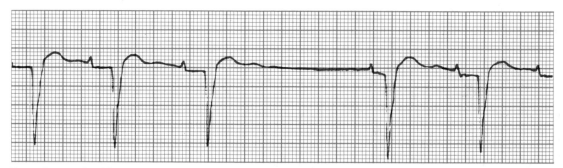

Practice strip 10

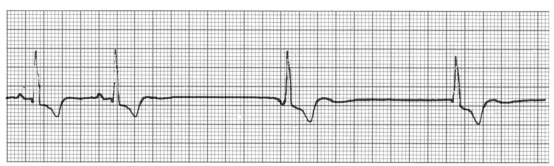

Practice strip 11

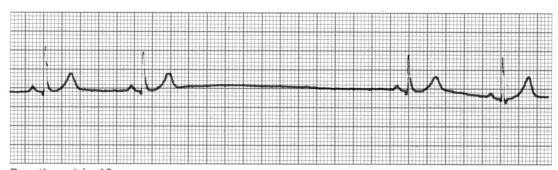

Practice strip 12

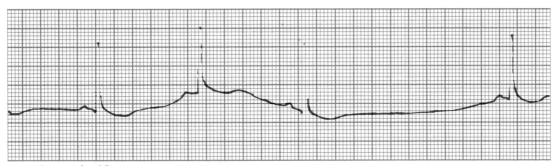

Practice strip 13

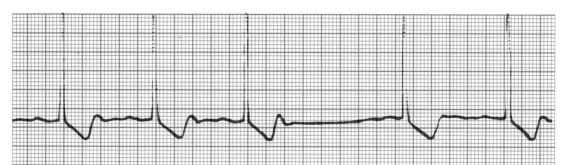

Practice strip 14

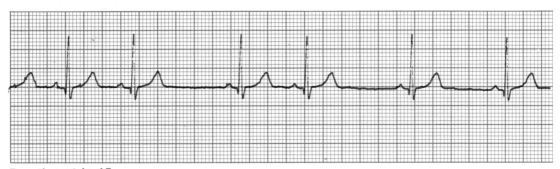

Practice strip 15

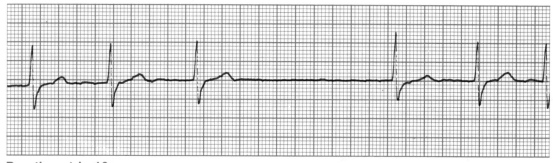

Practice strip 16

PRACTICE ECG STRIP ANSWERS

1. Sinus rhythm and APCs in trigeminy
2. Sinus rhythm and SA block Mobitz with two junctional escape beats
3. Sinus rhythm and SA block Mobitz
4. Sinus bradycardia with three isolated APCs, two with aberration
5. Sinus rhythm with SA block Wenckebach
6. Sinus rhythm with SA block Mobitz
7. Marked sinus bradycardia
8. Sinus bradycardia with SA block Mobitz
9. Sinus rhythm with a nonconducted APC and one isolated APC
10. Sinus rhythm with first degree AV block and SA block Mobitz with a junctional escape beat terminating the pause
11. Sinus rhythm with SA block and two junctional escape beats
12. Sinus bradycardia with SA block Mobitz
13. Sinus bradycardia with SA block Mobitz
14. Sinus bradycardia with first degree AV block and a nonconducted APC
15. Sinus arrhythmia
16. Atrial fibrillation with high grade AV block

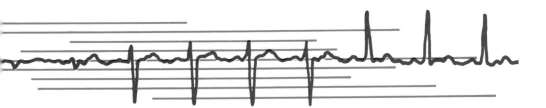

Chapter 12

PACEMAKER RHYTHMS

A pacemaker is an electrical device that is either temporarily inserted in a patient during an emergency or permanently implanted under the skin, usually in the chest wall. The pacemaker supplies the heart with the necessary electrical stimuli to enable it to depolarize and then contract when its own electrical conduction system no longer functions correctly and reliably.

NORMAL PACEMAKER FUNCTION

The pacemaker's electrical stimuli are recorded on an ECG strip as a *pacemaker spike*. Both the atria and the ventricles can be paced, individually or in combination, and when they respond to the pacemaker spike with a corresponding P wave or QRS complex, the pacemaker is said to *capture* the chamber.

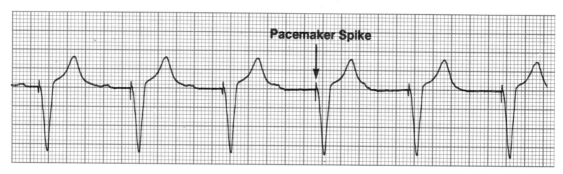

The atria are in sinus rhythm, and a ventricular pacemaker is firing at 60 beats per minute. The ventricles are completely controlled, or captured, by the electronic pacemaker stimuli. Sinus P waves have no relationship to the QRS complexes.

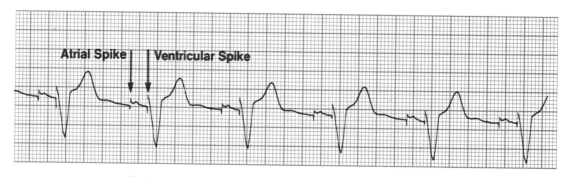

Both the atria and ventricles are being paced and are under the control of electronic pacemaker stimuli.

The most commonly used pacemakers today work in either the *inhibited mode* or the *triggered mode*. The inhibited pacemaker fires only when the heart rate goes below a determined level and so it works in a *demand mode*. The pacemaker's electronic circuitry is capable of *sensing* a spontaneous beat and temporarily turning off until needed again. The triggered pacemaker discharges after the onset of a spontaneous beat, but it plays no role in depolarization. Its spike only demonstrates a functioning pacemaker. But when the spontaneous rhythm falls below a specific rate, the triggered pacemaker assumes a fixed rate.

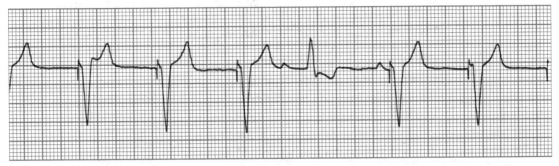

A ventricular inhibited pacemaker is firing at 70 beats per minute. A spontaneous sinus beat with first degree AV block is sensed, and the pacemaker does not fire. The pacemaker resumes its pacing function again when the heart rate becomes lower than the programmed pacemaker rate.

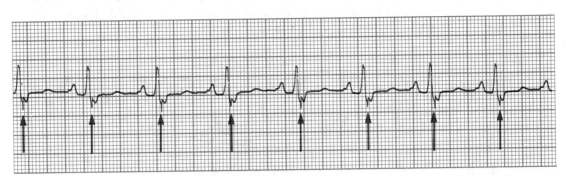

A ventricular triggered pacemaker showing pacemaker spikes (*arrows*) superimposed on spontaneous QRS complexes, demonstrating a functioning pacemaker. If the spontaneous heart rate falls below the programmed rate of the pacemaker, the pacemaker will fire at a fixed rate.

PACEMAKER RHYTHMS

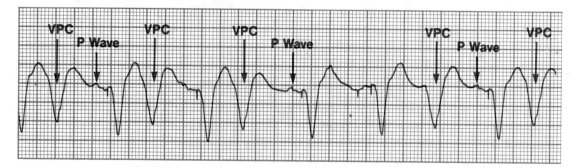

An atrial and ventricular inhibited pacemaker. The sensing function of the pacemaker is evidenced by the facts that both spontaneous P waves inhibit the atrial pacer and that VPCs inhibit the ventricular pacemaker.

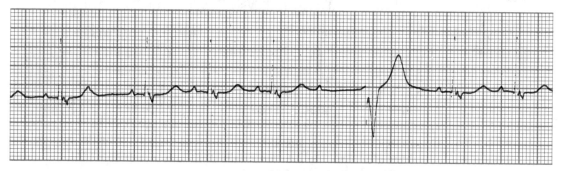

Sinus rhythm with one nonconducted APC and second degree AV block and the proper function of a ventricular inhibited pacemaker terminating the pause caused by the AV block

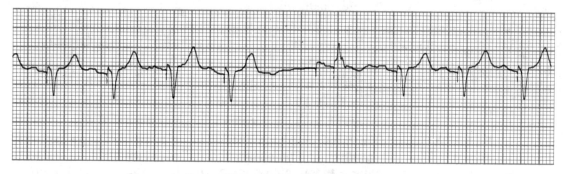

Sinus rhythm with probable SA block and a pause terminated by the proper function of an atrial and ventricular inhibited pacemaker

HOW TO QUICKLY AND ACCURATELY MASTER ARRHYTHMIA INTERPRETATION

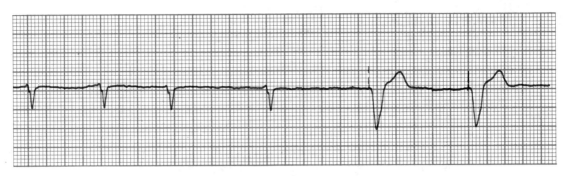

Atrial fibrillation and a ventricular inhibited pacemaker firing at a rate slightly below 60 beats per minute

There are different types of pacemakers on the market today, many of which are programmable when the need arises. It is not a goal of this book to discuss the modes of operation of the different types of pacemakers but rather to acquaint the student with common and easily recognizable pacemaker malfunctions in one-lead monitoring. Unless a pacemaker's programmed settings are known, there is no way to know whether it is functioning accurately or malfunctioning, except for the most obvious abnormalities. Those obvious malfunctions, which require no knowledge of the pacemaker's settings, are discussed and demonstrated in this chapter.

PACEMAKER MALFUNCTION

Failure to Sense

Failure to sense occurs when an inhibited pacemaker does not recognize a spontaneous beat and therefore does not inhibit its action, but continues to fire according to its preset rhythm. These additional spikes can cause ventricular depolarizations that will actually double the heart rate or may cause ventricular tachyarrhythmias if they are too premature.

A pacemaker can be programmed to override its inhibited action and fire continuously, simulating a failure to sense. But during emergency monitoring, when apparent nonsensing occurs, especially on an intermittent basis, always assume that a pacemaker malfunction is present.

The following criterion is used for recognition of the pacemaker malfunction known as failure to sense:

1. Pacemaker spikes occur when the pacemaker should be inhibited by the presence of spontaneous beats.

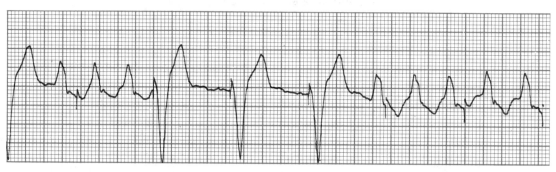

Ventricular inhibited pacemaker at 70 beats per minute firing at a fixed rate with no sensing function. Two runs of unifocal VPCs are not sensed as the pacemaker continues to fire. The pacemaker should remain inhibited when spontaneous beats occur.

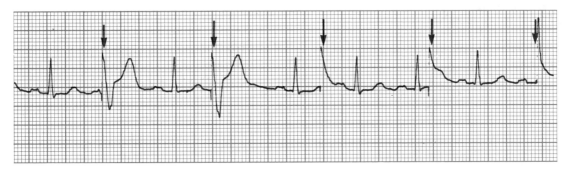

Sinus rhythm with a ventricular inhibited pacemaker that continues to fire at a fixed rate, offering no sensing capabilities and causing an accelerated heart rate. If the pacemaker spike falls outside the refractory period, the ventricles are captured, and a resulting QRS is inscribed on the ECG. If the pacemaker spike falls in the refractory period, no QRS complex follows the pacemaker spike. The pacemaker activity is indicated by the arrows.

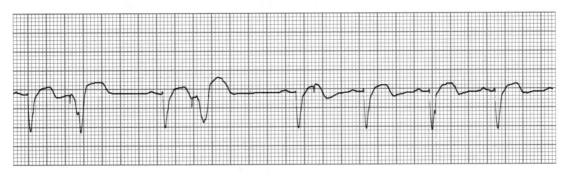

Sinus rhythm with intermittent nonsensing of a ventricular inhibited pacemaker. Three separate times the pacemaker does not sense the spontaneous sinus beats, as demonstrated by two inappropriate paced beats and one spike. The third pacer spike is not followed by a QRS complex because it falls in the refractory period.

Failure to Capture

During failure to capture, an electrical stimulus is emitted by the pacemaker, but it does not capture the chamber and cause depolarization or contraction. In a ventricular pacemaker with this malfunction, long ventricular pauses occur, or an escape rhythm may take over, controlling the heart rhythm.

The following criterion is used for recognition of the pacemaker malfunction known as failure to capture:

1. Pacemaker spikes occurring at a predetermined rate without the expected complexes following them. In malfunction of a ventricular pacemaker, long ventricular pauses or escape rhythms can occur.

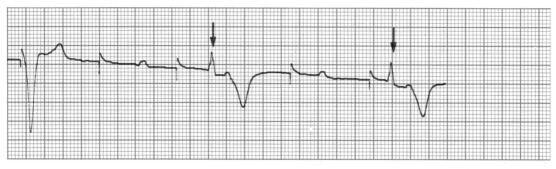

Intermittent failure of a ventricular pacemaker to capture the ventricles and record a QRS complex. A ventricular escape rhythm has taken over control of the ventricles. There are pacemaker spikes with no corresponding ventricular depolarizations recorded. The ventricular escape beats are indicated by the arrows.

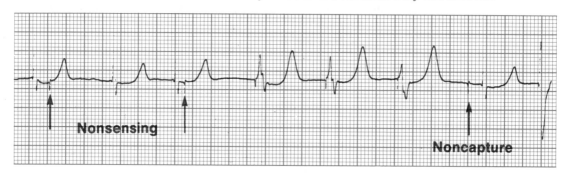

Intermittent ventricular inhibited pacemaker with probable atrial fibrillation as the underlying rhythm. There is intermittent failure to sense and failure to capture. The last beat of the strip is a VPC.

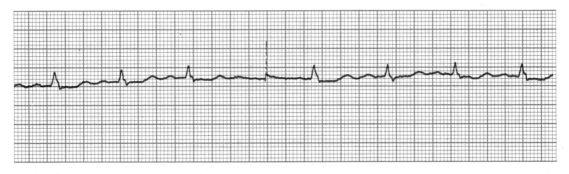

Sinus rhythm with first degree AV block and a pacemaker spike with no QRS complex following it, demonstrating a failure to capture the ventricles

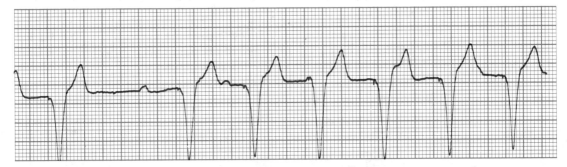

A ventricular pacemaker firing at 80 beats per minute with one episode of a pacemaker spike with no QRS complex following it, producing a ventricular pause. This demonstrates a failure to capture the ventricles.

DIFFERENTIAL DIAGNOSIS

Pacemaker spike or artifact?

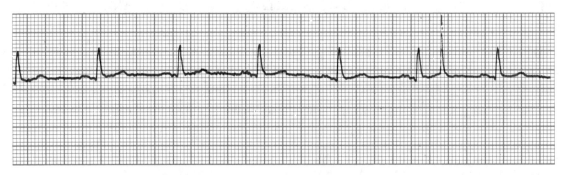

Sinus rhythm with artifact distorting the T wave. The questionable spike is too large to be considered a pacemaker spike. Without any other evidence of pacemaker activity a pacemaker is ruled out, and artifact is considered the correct interpretation.

Pacemaker spike or artifact?

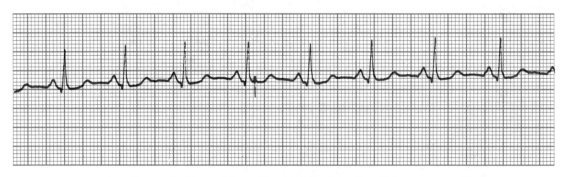

Sinus rhythm with artifact distorting the ST segment. Without any other evidence of pacemaker activity, the one spike is insufficient evidence for a pacemaker.

Pacemaker spike or artifact?

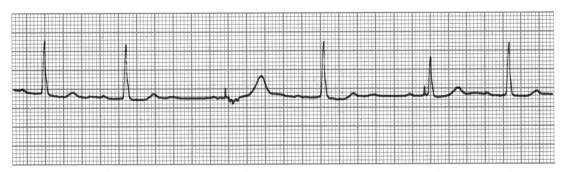

Sinus rhythm with first degree AV block and a ventricular inhibited pacemaker. A ventricular pause is terminated by a wide and bizarre QRS preceded by an apparent pacemaker spike. This could be a ventricular escape beat preceded by artifact, but the additional spike two beats to the right, followed by a QRS complex that appears to be a fusion beat between normal and pacemaker beats, confirms the interpretation of intermittent ventricular inhibited pacemaker.

Failure to sense or failure to capture?

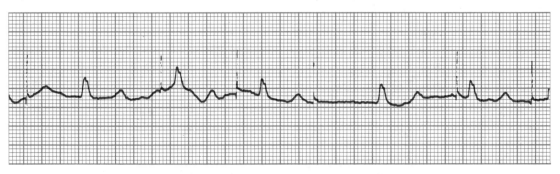

Atrial fibrillation with bundle branch block, failure to capture, and intermittent failure to sense. The pacemaker spikes never capture the ventricles and produces a QRS complex. The first and fourth spontaneous QRS complexes are sensed, and the pacemaker inhibits its action before firing again. The second, third, and fifth QRS complexes are not sensed and are followed by pacemaker spikes as if the spontaneous beats had not occurred.

Proper pacemaker function or malfunction

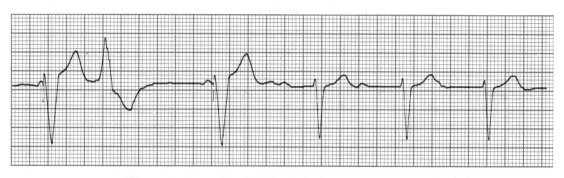

Sinus rhythm with AV block is present, and proper function of a ventricular inhibited pacemaker is noted as it senses both the sinus rhythm and the isolated VPC.

PRACTICE ECG STRIPS

I have purposely included artifact in some of the ECG strips to simulate the types of strips you might expect to find in the field. Eyeball the PR and QRS intervals for normal or abnormal intervals rather than exact measurements. Estimate the rate, identify the rhythm, and label any arrhythmias present.

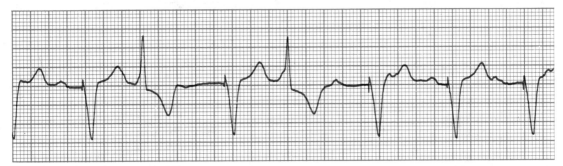

Practice strip 1

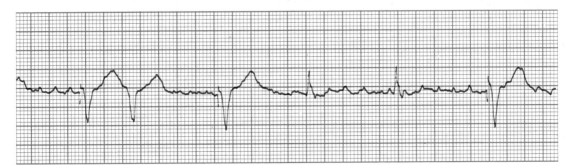

Practice strip 2

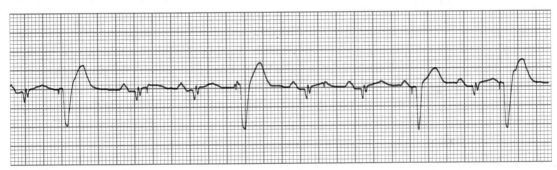

Practice strip 3

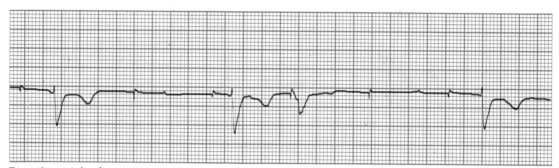

Practice strip 4

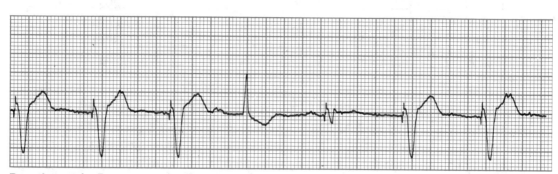

Practice strip 5

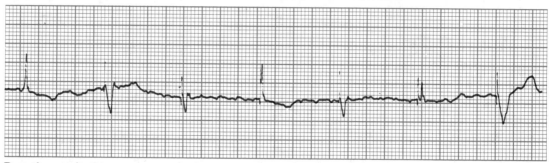

Practice strip 6

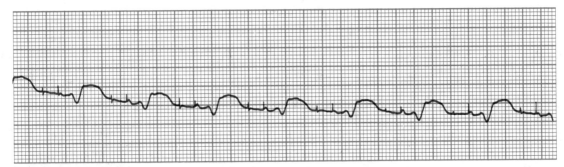

Practice strip 7

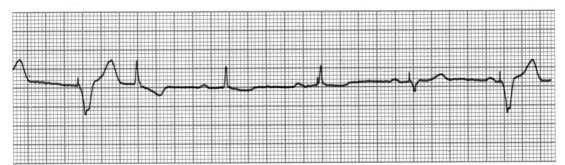

Practice strip 8

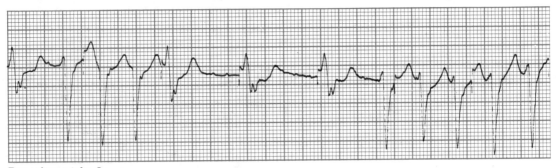

Practice strip 9

PACEMAKER RHYTHMS

233

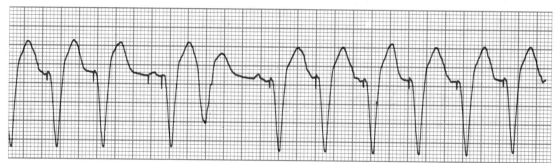

Practice strip 10

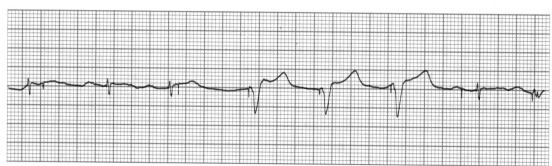

Practice strip 11

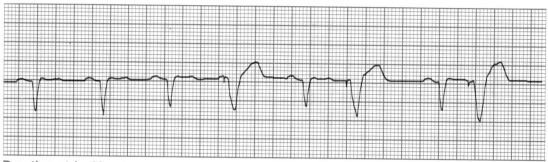

Practice strip 12

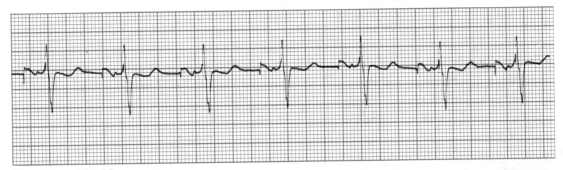

Practice strip 13

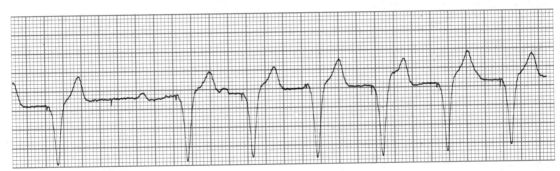

Practice strip 14

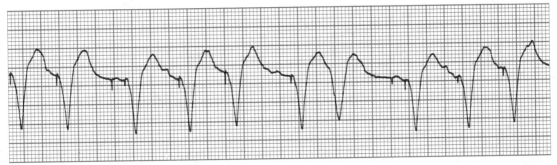

Practice strip 15

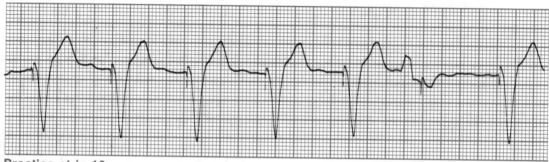

Practice strip 16

PRACTICE ECG STRIP ANSWERS

1. Proper function of a ventricular inhibited pacemaker. The VPCs are properly sensed.

2. Atrial fibrillation with proper function of a ventricular inhibited pacemaker and one VPC

3. Sinus rhythm with nonsensing of a ventricular inhibited pacemaker

4. Intermittent nonsensing and noncapture of a ventricular inhibited pacemaker and a ventricular escape rhythm

5. Sinus rhythm with first degree AV block and a properly functioning ventricular inhibited pacemaker and one fusion beat

6. Atrial fibrillation and proper function of a ventricular inhibited pacemaker with fusion beats

7. Atrial and ventricular pacemaker demonstrating failure to capture the atria

8. Sinus bradycardia with first degree AV block and proper function of a ventricular inhibited pacemaker with fusion beats

9. Ventricular pacemaker with failure to sense during runs of VPCs

10. Proper function of an atrial and ventricular inhibited pacemaker with one VPC

11. Sinus rhythm with a ventricular inhibited pacemaker demonstrating intermittent failure to sense and capture

12. Sinus rhythm with a ventricular inhibited pacemaker demonstrating a failure to sense

13. Atrial pacemaker with proper function at 70 beats per minute

14. Ventricular pacemaker with intermittent failure to capture

15. Atrial and ventricular inhibited pacemaker functioning properly with one VPC

16. Ventricular pacemaker that does not sense a VPC

Chapter 13

HOW TO MAKE RAPID AND ACCURATE INTERPRETATIONS IN THE FIELD

Working in the field requires quick and accurate interpretations of an ECG strip. The entire strip must be scanned and evaluated for initial impressions. The strip should then be checked for regularity of rhythm; presence, absence, or variation of P waves, PR intervals, and QRS complexes; and routine measurements. After the first careful observations, you should begin ruling out or confirming the initial impressions until you arrive at the correct diagnosis.

The following ECGs are presented for evaluation, and the analysis of each interpretation follows the protocol given above.

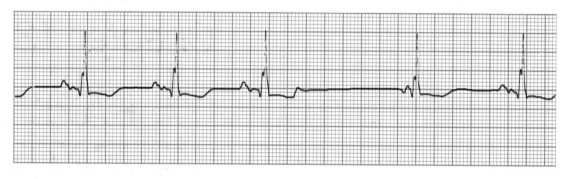

Initial impressions. (1) SA block, (2) nonconducted APC, or (3) sinus arrhythmia

Regular rhythm? Yes, except for a ventricular pause

P waves present? Yes

PR interval constant? Yes, except for one P wave that is inverted and has a shorter PR interval

PR and QRS intervals normal? QRS wide

Final interpretation. On examination of the T wave preceding the ventricular pause, a definite P wave is noted superimposed on its ascending limb. Because it is an early P wave, a nonconducted APC is diagnosed. The pause is terminated by a junctional escape beat. Sinus rhythm with bundle branch block is present.

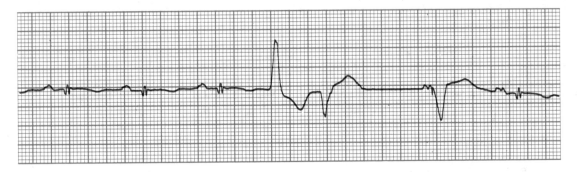

Initial impressions. Sinus rhythm with first degree AV block and (1) VPCs with a ventricular escape beat, (2) VPCs and a pacemaker beat, or (3) APCs with aberration followed by either a paced beat or a ventricular escape beat

Regular rhythm? No. Premature beats are present, and a late beat terminates a pause.

P waves present? Yes, but not on all beats

PR interval constant? Yes, with sinus beats

PR and QRS intervals normal? PR long

Final interpretation. Sinus rhythm with first degree AV block is easy to diagnose in this strip. The early beats are wide and bizarre and are not preceded by ectopic P waves. This rules out aberration and verifies the diagnosis of a pair of multifocal VPCs. A ventricular escape beat seems to terminate the pause, but on careful inspection a pacemaker spike is seen preceding the wide and bizarre QRS, confirming the diagnosis of a ventricular inhibited pacemaker.

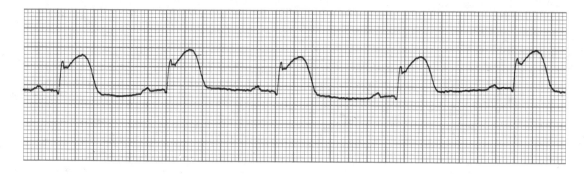

Initial impressions. (1) Sinus rhythm with first degree AV block and a bundle branch block or (2) sinus rhythm with first degree AV block

Regular rhythm? Yes

P waves present? Yes

PR interval constant? Yes

PR and QRS intervals normal? PR long

Final interpretation. On first examination the QRS appears wide and bizarre and seems to fit the criteria for bundle branch block. Actually, however, the QRS is of normal duration and the ST segment and T wave are elevated off the isoelectric line because of an acute infarction, giving the appearance of a widened QRS. Sinus rhythm with first degree AV block is present.

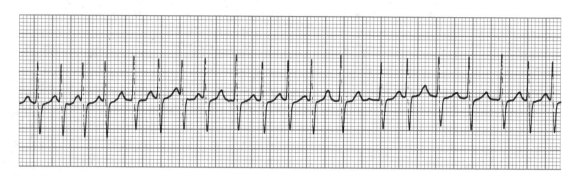

Initial impressions. (1) Atrial fibrillation, (2) atrial flutter, (3) junctional tachycardia, or (4) atrial tachycardia

Regular rhythm? Appears regular because of the rapid ventricular rate, but on close examination it is not. Careful examinations are mandatory for accurate interpretations.

P waves present? No

PR interval constant? None

PR and QRS intervals normal? Yes

Final interpretation. No ectopic atrial waves are seen, and because of the irregular ventricular response, atrial fibrillation is the correct interpretation.

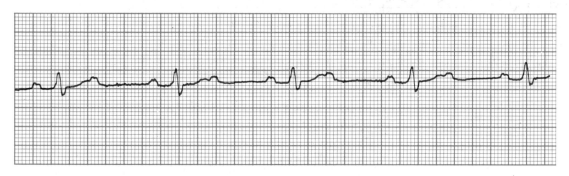

Initial impressions. Sinus rhythm with first degree AV block and bundle branch block and (1) nonconducted APCs in bigeminy or (2) second degree AV block Mobitz

Regular rhythm? P-P and R-R cycles are regular

P waves present? Yes, two P waves for each QRS. An additional P wave is superimposed on the previous T wave

PR interval constant? Yes

PR and QRS intervals normal? PR long and QRS wide

Final interpretation. On careful examination, there are definitely P waves hidden in all the T waves, and the P-P cycle appears regular, with no early beats. This confirms the interpretation of second degree AV block Mobitz and bundle branch block with AV block and rules out the possibility of nonconducted APCs.

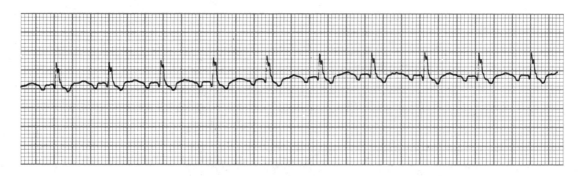

Initial impressions. (1) PAT with 2 : 1 block, (2) atrial flutter with 2 : 1 block, or (3) junctional tachycardia

Regular rhythm? P-P and R-R cycles are regular

P waves present? Inverted P waves or F waves are present, all with the same configuration. There are two atrial waves for each QRS complex

PR interval constant? Yes

PR and QRS intervals normal? Yes

Final interpretation. The atrial rate is approximately 200 per minute—an additional P wave occurring in the T wave of the previous beat. The atrial rhythm is regular and because of the rate fits the criteria for PAT with 2 : 1 block. There are two P waves for each QRS complex. If the atrial rate were 220 or above, the diagnosis of atrial flutter with 2 : 1 block would apply. Although this appears to be atrial flutter, the atrial rate rules that out. Initially, it appears as if a junctional tachycardia is present because of the apparent inverted P waves, but there are additional atrial waves in the preceding T waves, and junctional tachycardia is ruled out.

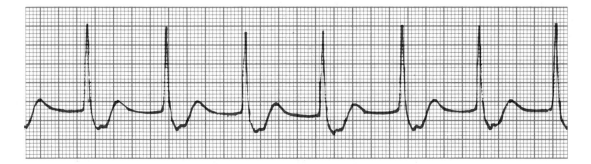

Initial impressions. Junctional rhythm

Regular rhythm? Yes

P waves present? Yes, inverted P waves following each QRS in the T wave

PR interval constant? None

PR and QR intervals normal? Yes

Final interpretation. Accelerated junctional rhythm

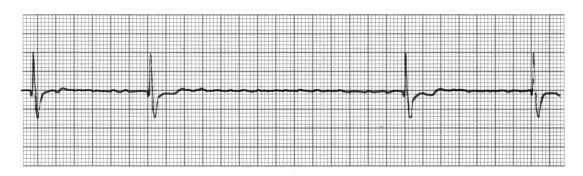

Initial impressions. Atrial fibrillation

Regular rhythm? No, irregular ventricular response

P waves present? No. Fibrillatory waves are present.

PR interval constant? None

PR and QRS interval normal? Yes

Final interpretation. The diagnosis of atrial fibrillation was not difficult because of the presence of fibrillatory waves and the irregular ventricular response. The ventricular pauses are long enough to be attributable to high grade AV block.

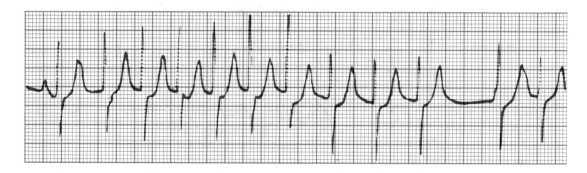

Initial impressions. (1) Atrial tachycardia, (2) multifocal atrial tachycardia, or (3) atrial fibrillation

Regular rhythm? No

P waves present? A few P waves are noted.

PR interval constant? No

PR and QRS intervals normal? Yes

Final interpretation. The first beat is a sinus beat. A run of probable atrial tachycardia follows. The first APC is preceded by a distorted T wave, and an ectopic P wave is probably superimposed on it. The run of APCs is then followed by a pause, which is terminated by a junctional escape beat. Multifocal atrial tachycardia is ruled out because of the absence of various ectopic P waves and PR intervals, and atrial fibrillation is not considered because of the apparent initial ectopic P wave beginning the atrial tachycardia.

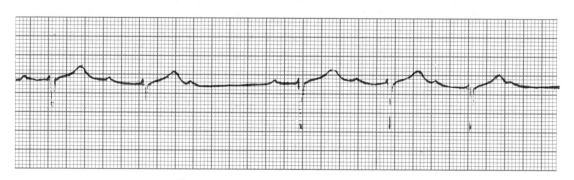

Initial impressions. (1) Second degree AV block Wenckebach, (2) second degree AV block Mobitz, or (3) nonconducted APCs

Regular rhythm? Atrial rate regular, ventricular rate irregular

P waves present? Yes

PR interval constant? PR interval varies

PR and QRS intervals normal? PR interval long

Final interpretation. Nonconducted APCs are immediately ruled out because the atrial rate is regular, with no early beats. The PR interval becomes progressively longer with each beat until a P wave is not conducted and a ventricular pause occurs. The cycle then repeats itself. This strip demonstrates sinus rhythm with first degree AV block and second degree AV block Wenckebach.

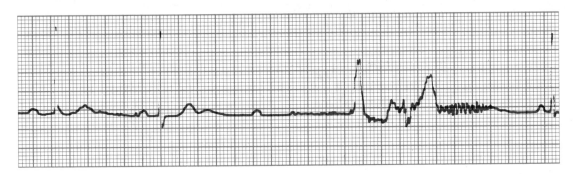

Initial impressions. (1) Second degree AV block Mobitz or (2) complete AV block

Regular rhythm? The first part of the strip shows a regular P-wave cycle that is interrupted by wide and bizarre QRS complexes and then reverts back to a regular cycle.

P waves present? Yes

PR interval constant? Yes, on the first two beats

PR and QRS intervals normal? PR interval long

Final interpretation. The lone sinus P wave occurring on time and not followed by a QRS substantiates the diagnosis of second degree AV block Mobitz. Complete AV block is ruled out because of the presence of sinus rhythm and normal conduction in both the beginning and the end of the strip. The ventricular pause is terminated by a ventricular escape beat because it occurs later than the normal R-R cycle, and is immediately followed by an early, wide, bizarre QRS, representing a VPC. Often, after a long ventricular pause, the PR intervals of the next sinus beats are normally slightly shorter.

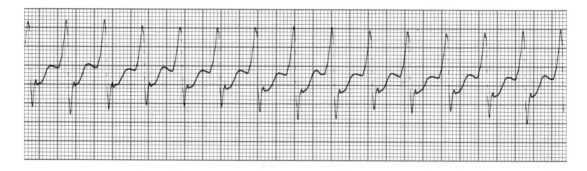

Initial impressions. (1) Ventricular tachycardia or (2) junctional tachy-cardia with bundle branch block

Regular rhythm? Yes

P waves present? No

PR interval constant? None

PR and QRS intervals normal? QRS complexes are wide.

Final interpretation. In this strip there is no way to differentiate the two initial impressions. Unless there is evidence of a predisposing bundle branch block, always assume that a ventricular tachycardia is present

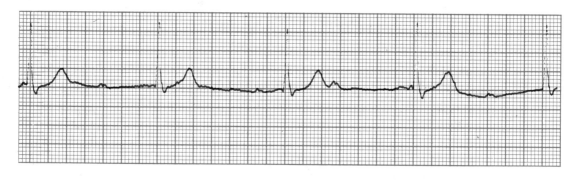

Initial impressions. (1) Second degree AV block Wenckebach or (2) complete AV block

Regular rhythm? P-P and R-R cycles are regular.

P waves present? Yes

PR interval constant? Varies

PR and QRS intervals normal? The PR varies, and the QRS com-plexes are wide.

Final interpretation. Although the PR interval does vary, none of the P waves ever conduct to the ventricles. The P-P cycle is regular but bears no relationship to the QRS complexes. The atria are under the control of sinus rhythm, and the ventricles are being paced by a ventricular escape rhythm in complete AV block. In second degree AV block Wenckebach with varying PR intervals, there would eventually be a nonconducted P wave followed by a pause, which does not occur in this strip.

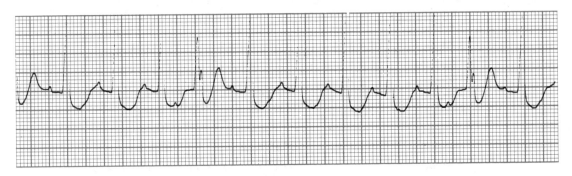

Initial impressions. Sinus tachycardia with (1) APCs with aberration, (2) VPCs, or (3) intermittent bundle branch block

Regular rhythm? Yes, except for the two wide and bizarre beats

P waves present? Yes

PR interval constant? Yes, in sinus beats

PR and QRS intervals normal? Yes

Final interpretation. Each early, wide, bizarre beat is clearly preceded by an ectopic P wave, demonstrating APCs with aberration. If this were an intermittent bundle branch block, the P-P cycle would be regular with no early beats. Just the QRS would intermittently widen.

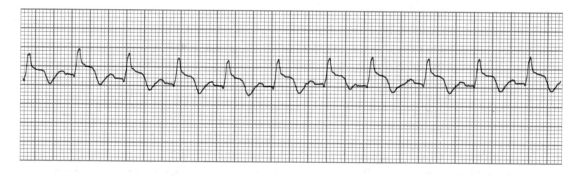

Initial impressions. (1) Ventricular tachycardia, (2) sinus tachycardia, or (3) sinus tachycardia with bundle branch block

Regular rhythm? Yes

P waves present? Yes

PR interval constant? Yes

PR and QRS intervals normal? Yes

Final interpretation. Although the QRS complex appears widened, it is of normal duration and is being disfigured by the marked ST elevation of acute infarction. Sinus P waves appear to follow immediately after each T wave, and this would confirm the diagnosis of sinus tachycardia with one isolated APC.

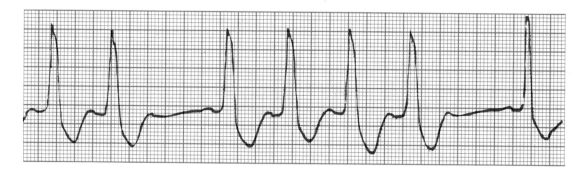

Initial impressions. (1) Runs of APCs, (2) SA block, (3) nonconducted APCs, or (4) runs of VPCs

Regular rhythm? No

P waves present? Yes

PR interval constant? On two beats

PR and QRS intervals normal? QRS wide

Final interpretation. The two beats with constant PR intervals are sinus beats and follow the ventricular pauses. Because both sinus beats have a widened QRS complex, bundle branch block is present. With the establishment of bundle branch block as the cause of the wide QRS complexes, the apparent early beats are not VPCs but simply APCs or JPCs. Ventricular pauses follow each burst of supraventricular premature beats as the sinus node prepares to resume its pacing cycle.

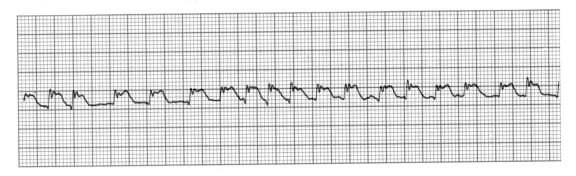

Initial impressions. (1) Atrial fibrillation, (2) atrial fibrillation with bundle branch block, or (3) ventricular tachycardia

Regular rhythm? No. Ventricular response rapid and irregular.

P waves present? Not apparent

PR interval constant? None

PR and QRS intervals normal? Yes

Final interpretation. Although the ventricular response is not regular, a widened QRS and a rapid rate are always clues to ventricular tachycardia. But on close examination it is apparent that the QRS is not actually widened but only distorted by an elevated ST segment of an acute infarction. With the irregular ventricular response, a normal QRS duration, and the absence of P waves, the interpretation of atrial fibrillation with a rapid ventricular response is correct.

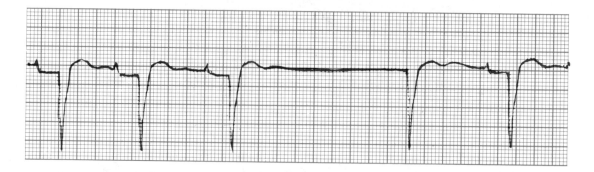

Initial impressions. (1) Nonconducted APC, (2) sinus arrhythmia, or (3) SA block

Regular rhythm? Yes, except for a ventricular pause

P waves present? Yes

PR interval constant? Yes, except for the beat following the pause (no PR present)

PR and QRS intervals normal? PR long and QRS wide

Final interpretation. There is no visible ectopic P wave buried in the T wave before the ventricular pause, ruling out a nonconducted APC. The pause is too long and too abrupt to be sinus arrhythmia, and sinus arrhythmia is usually not terminated by a junctional escape beat. Sinus rhythm with first degree AV block and bundle branch block with second degree SA block Mobitz is the arrhythmia present in this strip. The ventricular pause is terminated by a junctional escape beat.

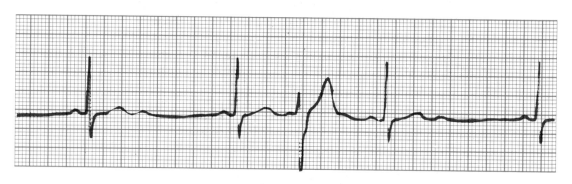

Initial impressions. (1) Nonconducted APCs with one APC with aberration, (2) second degree AV block Mobitz and one VPC, (3) sinus bradycardia with one VPC followed by one APC, or (4) sinus bradycardia with an interpolated VPC

Regular rhythm? Yes. P-P and R-R cycles are regular.

P waves present? Yes

PR interval constant? Yes

PR and QRS intervals normal? Yes

Final interpretation. Second degree AV block Mobitz is ruled out because the questionable P waves following each T wave are actually U waves and do not occur in time to make a regular P-P cycle. The possibility of nonconducted APCs is also discounted because if the U waves were really early APCs, they should have been conducted, for they fall well outside the refractory period. So sinus bradycardia is present, and all the sinus beats fall exactly on time, including the P wave and QRS immediately following the VPC. The interpretation is sinus bradycardia with one interpolated VPC that does not interrupt the sinus cycle at all.

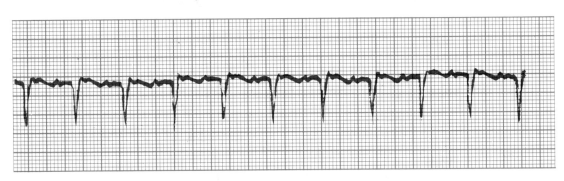

Initial impressions. (1) Atrial flutter, (2) PAT with block, or (3) sinus tachycardia with first degree AV block

Regular rhythm? Yes

P waves present? Yes, two for each QRS. The initial part of each T wave is distorted by the additional P wave.

PR interval constant? Yes

PR and QRS intervals normal? Yes

Final interpretation. There are two P waves for each QRS, and the atrial rate is approximately 200 per minute. This fits the criteria for PAT with 2:1 block.

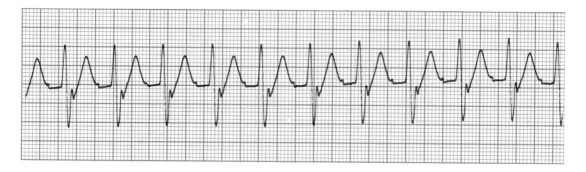

Initial impressions. (1) Ventricular tachycardia or (2) sinus tachycardia with bundle branch block.

Regular rhythm? Yes

P waves present? Tiny P waves precede each QRS complex.

PR interval constant? Yes

PR and QRS intervals normal? QRS wide

Final interpretation. Sinus tachycardia with bundle branch block. The presence of the sinus P waves with a constant PR interval rules out the possibility of ventricular tachycardia.

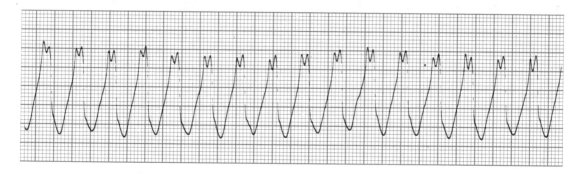

Initial impressions. (1) Ventricular tachycardia or (2) supraventricular tachycardia with bundle branch block or aberration

Regular rhythm? Yes

P waves present? No

PR interval constant? None

PR and QRS intervals normal? QRS wide

Final interpretation. Because of the absence of P waves and the widened QRS complex, the interpretation of ventricular tachycardia is correct.

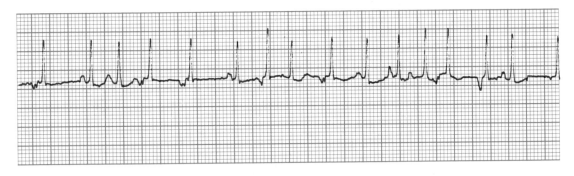

Initial impressions. (1) Mulitfocal atrial tachycardia, (2) atrial fibrillation, or (3) runs of APCs

Regular rhythm? No

P waves present? Yes—many different configurations

PR interval constant? No

PR and QRS intervals normal? Yes

Final interpretation. The variation in the PR intervals and the configurations of the P waves confirm the diagnosis of multifocal atrial tachycardia. The presence of P waves rules out atrial fibrillation, and because of the variety of multifocal APCs the diagnosis simply of runs of APCs, although correct, is not sufficiently specific.

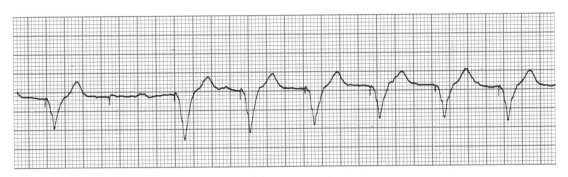

Initial impressions. Pacemaker failure: (1) nonsensing, (2) noncapture, or (3) nonsensing and noncapture

Regular rhythm? Yes, except for a ventricular pause

P waves present? Yes, a few

PR interval constant? No

PR and QRS intervals normal? QRS wide

Final interpretation. A ventricular pacemaker is present, with the second spike failing to elicit a response and demonstrating a failure to capture the ventricles, producing a ventricular pause

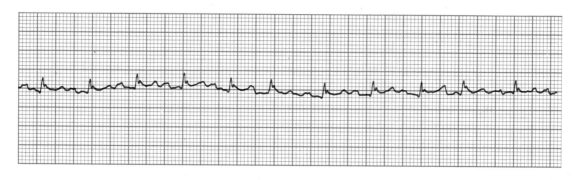

Initial impressions. (1) Atrial flutter, (2) sinus tachycardia with APCs, (3) multifocal atrial tachycardia, or (4) PAT with block

Regular rhythm? No

P waves present? Yes

PR interval constant? Complexes are small, and artifact is present, but the PR interval appears constant.

PR and QRS intervals normal? PR is long

Final interpretation. This is a difficult strip because artifact is present and the complexes are so tiny. No regular pattern for flutter waves can be discerned. The R-R cycle appears regular for most of the strip, but there are intermittent short R-R cycles followed by longer ones, suggesting premature beats. On close inspection the short R-R cycles are preceded by ectopic P waves buried in the T waves of the preceding beats, confirming the diagnosis of sinus tachycardia with first degree AV block and two isolated APCs.

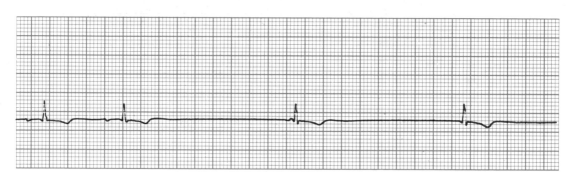

Initial impressions. (1) SA block or (2) sinus arrhythmia

Regular rhythm? No

P waves present? Yes, on the first three beats

PR interval constant? On the first two beats

PR and QRS intervals normal? Yes

Final interpretation. Sinus rhythm is present. Long ventricular pauses, with the sudden absence of the original sinus P waves, represents SA block. Sinus arrhythmia usually presents a more gradual variation in the R-R cycle and is usually not terminated by junctional escape beats as occur in this strip.

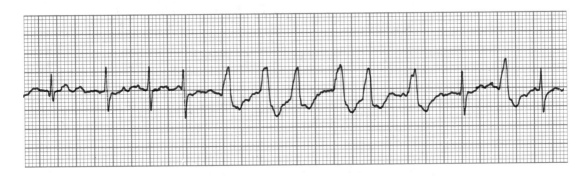

Initial impressions. (1) Atrial fibrillation with runs of ventricular tachycardia or (2) atrial fibrillation with aberrant beats

Regular rhythm? No

P waves present? No

PR interval constant? None

PR and QRS intervals normal? Intermittent wide and bizarre beats

Final interpretation. Because the underlying rhythm is atrial fibrillation with varying R-R cycles, aberration must be a consideration. Because the run of wide beats also has an irregular R-R cycle, just like the underlying rhythm, the wide beats are probably aberrant beats and not VPCs as initially suspected.

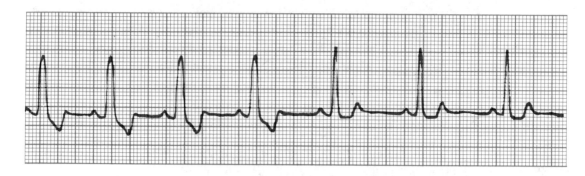

Initial impressions. (1) Runs of VPCs, (2) runs of APCs with aberration, or (3) intermittent bundle branch block

Regular rhythm? Yes

P waves present? Yes

PR interval constant? Yes

PR and QRS intervals normal? QRS widens intermittently.

Final interpretation. The P-P cycle and the PR interval are constant throughout the strip. Only the QRS width changes. VPCs and APCs are ruled out because there are no early beats, and constant PR intervals precede each wide beat. Sinus rhythm with intermittent bundle branch block is the correct interpretation, and as the rate slows down ever so slightly, the bundle branch block disappears and a normal QRS interval appears.

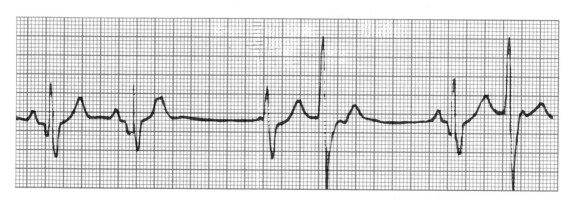

Initial impressions. (1) Nonconducted APC and VPCs or (2) SA block and VPCs

Regular rhythm? No, pauses and early beats

P waves present? Yes

PR interval constant? Yes, on the sinus beats

PR and QRS intervals normal? QRS wide

Final interpretation. The ventricular pause is caused by a nonconducted APC sitting right on top of the previous T wave and distorting it. The ectopic P wave is too obvious to cause any confusion. The pause is terminated by a junctional escape beat and then followed by two isolated, unifocal VPCs. A bundle branch block is also present.

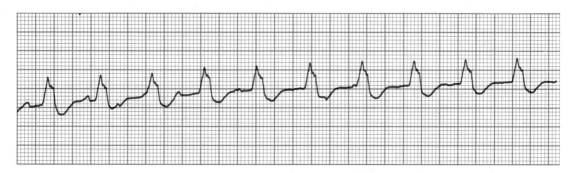

Initial impressions. (1) Ventricular tachycardia or (2) sinus tachycardia with bundle branch block

Regular rhythm? Yes

P waves present? Yes

PR interval constant? No

PR and QRS intervals normal? QRS wide

Final interpretation. Although P waves are present, the PR interval varies. Regular conduction is not occurring, so there is no bundle branch block. AV dissociation is present between the atria and the ventricles. The atria are controlled by either an ectopic supraventricular rhythm or sinus tachycardia, and the ventricles are controlled by a run of ventricular tachycardia.

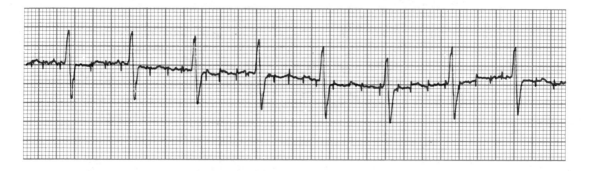

Initial impressions. (1) Malfunctioning, rapid-firing pacemaker, (2) atrial flutter, or (3) artifact

Regular rhythm? The ventricular rate is regular, but the atrial rate is not.

P waves present? No

PR interval constant? None

PR and QRS intervals normal? QRS wide

Final interpretation. Because the atrial rate is irregular, atrial flutter and a malfunctioning runaway pacemaker have been ruled out. Even though a pacemaker may malfunction and fire rapidly, it would usually do so at a set rate. The rhythm is probably sinus with bundle branch block and excessive artifact. The clue that artifact is present is the lack of regularity to the markings and the variation in configurations. This patient had muscle movement during the recording, which simulated an arrhythmia.

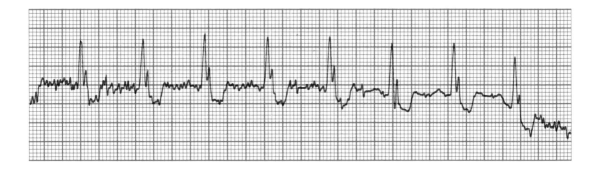

Initial impressions. Gross artifact

Regular rhythm? Appears to be regular

P wave present? Two are clearly noted.

PR interval constant? Constant in both beats seen

PR and QRS intervals normal? QRS wide

Final interpretation. Even though gross artifact distorts this ECG, it is obvious that the QRS is widened, and sinus P waves can be seen in front of two of the widened QRS complexes, leading to the probability of sinus rhythm with bundle branch block.

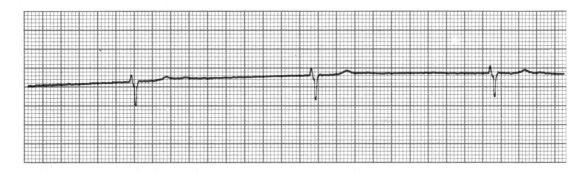

Initial impressions. (1) Junctional escape rhythm

Regular rhythm? Yes

P waves present? No

PR interval constant? None

PR and QRS intervals normal? Yes

Final interpretation. Junctional escape rhythm with atrial standstill— no atrial activity is noted. The ventricular rate is extremely low at 35 beats per minute.

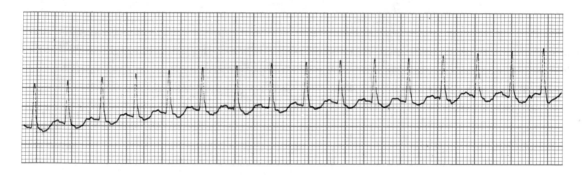

Initial impressions. (1) Atrial tachycardia, (2) atrial flutter with 2 : 1 block (3) junctional tachycardia, or (4) atrial fibrillation with rapid ventricular response.

Regular rhythm? Yes

P waves present? Possibly

PR interval constant? Not apparent

PR and QRS intervals normal? Yes

Final interpretation. Atrial activity appears to occur before each QRS complex. It could represent an atrial tachycardia or one of two flutter waves preceding each QRS. Because of the inability to make a clear distinction, the interpretation of supraventricular tachycardia would be appropriate at this time.

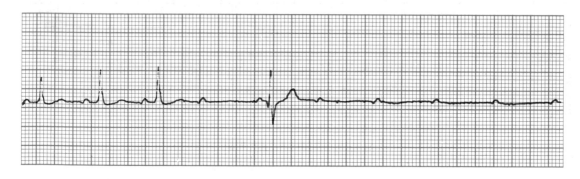

Initial impressions. (1) AV block

Regular rhythm? The atrial rhythm is regular. The ventricular rhythm disappears.

P waves present? Yes

PR interval constant? Yes, on the first three beats

PR and QRS intervals normal? Yes

Final interpretation. Sinus rhythm with complete AV block and a long run of sinus P waves with only one junctional escape beat occurring during the first two seconds of ventricular asystole. An escape mechanism took over pacing the ventricles after 40 seconds, and a pacemaker was inserted.

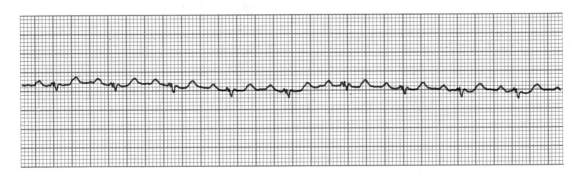

Initial impressions. (1) Sinus tachycardia, (2) atrial flutter with 2:1 block, or (3) PAT with 2:1 block

Regular rhythm? Yes

P waves present? Yes

PR interval constant? Yes

PR and QRS intervals normal? Yes

Final interpretation. The P-P cycle is regular at approximately 100 beats per minute, confirming the diagnosis of sinus rhythm. The questionable additional P wave for each QRS complex is actually the T wave of the previous beat, for it does not arrive in sufficient time to produce a regular P-P cycle.

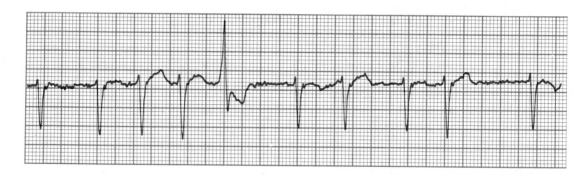

Initial impressions. (1) Atrial fibrillation with a VPC or (2) sinus rhythm with APCs and a VPC

Regular rhythm? No

P waves present? No

PR interval constant? None

PR and QRS intervals normal? Yes

Final interpretation. With the absence of P waves and the irregular ventricular response, the diagnosis of atrial fibrillation with one VPC is clear-cut.

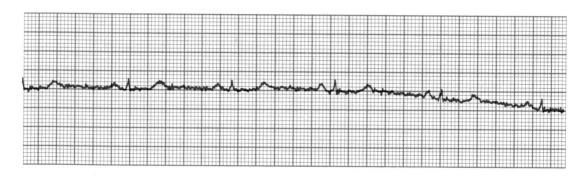

Initial impressions. (1) Complete AV block, (2) sinus bradycardia with first degree AV block, or (3) second degree AV block Mobitz

Regular rhythm? Yes

P waves present? Yes

PR interval constant? Yes

PR and QRS intervals normal? PR long

Final interpretation. Initially it appears as if there are additional P waves buried in the T waves, suggesting second degree AV block Mobitz. But the suspicious P waves are actually the T waves, which have a slightly different configuration from the sinus P waves and do not map out as part of a regular P-P cycle. This strip represents sinus bradycardia with first degree AV block.

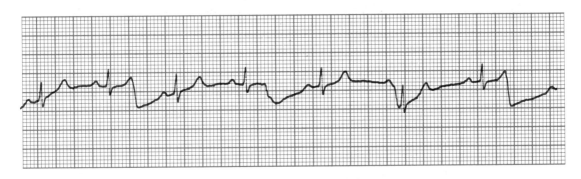

Initial impressions. (1) Second degree AV block Mobitz or (2) sinus rhythm

Regular rhythm? Yes

P waves present? Yes

PR interval constant? Yes

PR and QRS intervals normal? No

Final interpretation. Sinus rhythm is demonstrated in this strip. The T wave simulates a possible additional P wave for each QRS, suggesting second degree AV block Mobitz, but on close examination it does not map out as part of a regular P-P cycle.

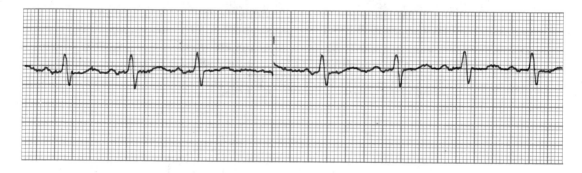

Initial impressions. Sinus rhythm with a pacemaker demonstrating (1) failure to capture or (2) failure to sense

Regular rhythm? Yes, except for ventricular pause

P waves present? Yes, on sinus beat

PR interval constant? Yes

PR and QRS intervals normal? Yes

Final interpretation. Sinus rhythm is present, and a ventricular pause occurs because the pacemaker spike failed to capture the ventricles.

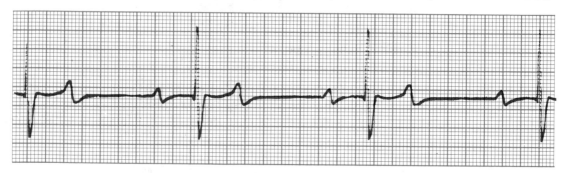

Initial impressions. (1) Complete AV block, (2) sinus bradycardia with first degree AV block, or (3) second degree AV block Mobitz.

Regular rhythm? P-P and R-R cycles are regular.

P waves present? Yes

PR interval constant? Yes

PR and QRS intervals normal? PR long and QRS wide

Final interpretation. Because of the constant PR intervals, complete AV block is immediately ruled out. A second P wave, with the same configuration as the obvious sinus P wave, appears in sufficient time to make the P-P cycle regular at 60 beats per minute. This strip indicates sinus rhythm with first degree AV block and bundle branch block with second degree AV block Mobitz.

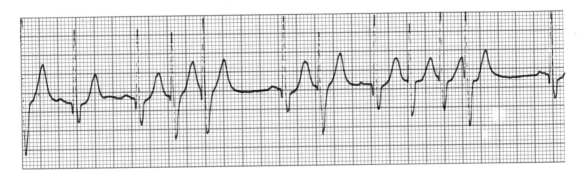

Initial impressions. Sinus rhythm with (1) JPCs or (2) VPCs

Regular rhythm? No

P waves present? Yes, on sinus beats

PR interval constant? Yes, on sinus beats

PR and QRS intervals normal? Yes

Final interpretation. Sinus rhythm is present with early beats isolated, in pairs, and three in a row. The early beats have almost the same configuration as the sinus beats, with no apparent widening, giving credence to the diagnosis of multiple APCs or JPCs rather than VPCs.

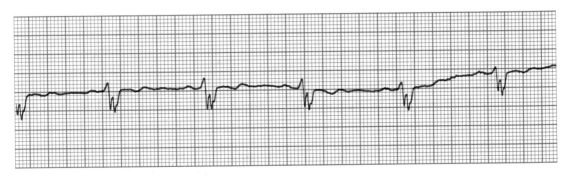

Initial impressions. (1) Atrial flutter, (2) atrial fibrillation, or (3) sinus bradycardia

Regular rhythm? Yes

P waves present? Yes

PR interval constant? Yes

PR and QRS intervals normal? QRS wide

Final interpretation. It appears as if multiple P or F waves may be present for each QRS, but on closer examination there is only one P wave for each QRS complex. The T waves and the appearance of U waves tend to resemble additional P waves. This strip is simply sinus bradycardia with a bundle branch block.

HOW TO MAKE RAPID AND ACCURATE INTERPRETATIONS IN THE FIELD

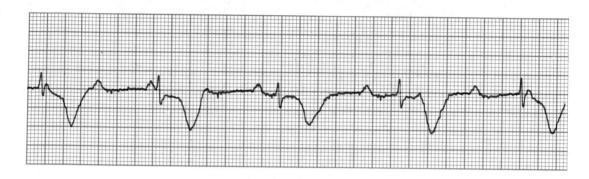

Initial impressions. (1) Complete AV block or (2) sinus bradycardia with AV dissociation

Regular rhythm? Yes

P waves present? Yes

PR interval constant? No

PR and QRS intervals normal? Yes

Final interpretation. Sinus bradycardia is immediately ruled out because careful examination shows multiple P waves for each QRS at a rate of approximately 100 beats per minute. Sinus rhythm is present with complete AV block and a junctional escape beat controlling the ventricles.

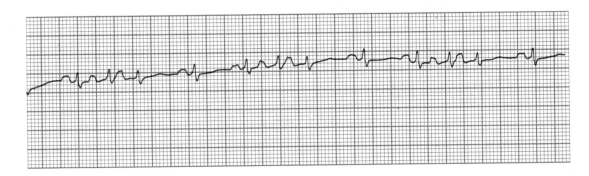

Initial impressions. (1) Multifocal atrial tachycardia, (2) second degree AV block Wenckebach, or (3) multiple APCs

Regular rhythm? No

P waves present? Yes

PR interval constant? Yes, on sinus beats

PR and QRS intervals normal? Yes

Final interpretation. There are clear sinus beats present throughout the strip, easily recognized because of the constant PR interval, and there are pairs of APCs present in trigeminy. Although the PR intervals of each pair of APCs become longer as in AV block Wenckebach, there is no evidence of dropped P waves.

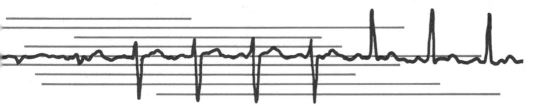

INDEX

INDEX

Aberration, 158–163. *See also* Wolff–Parkinson–White syndrome
  in atrial fibrillation, 159, 161–162
    vs atrial fibrillation with ventricular tachycardia, 257
  in atrial flutter, 159
    vs ventricular premature contractions, 168–169
  in atrial premature contractions, 159–162
    vs fusion beats, 168
    vs intermittent bundle branch block, 258
    sinus tachycardia with, 249
    vs ventricular inhibited pacemaker, 241
    vs VPC–APC combination, 167
  in atrial tachycardia, *vs* ventricular tachycardia, 169
  criteria for recognition of, 159
  definition of, 158
  differential diagnosis of, 167–169
  in junctional premature contractions, 159–160
  in junctional tachycardia, 163
  physiology of, 158
  in supraventricular premature beat, *vs* ventricular premature contractions, 167
  in supraventricular tachycardia, 162
  vs ventricular premature contractions, 158
  vs ventricular tachycardia, 158
Absolute refractory period, 10
Accelerated idioventricular rhythm, 136–137
Accelerated junctional rhythms. *See under* Junctional ectopic rhythms
AC interference, artifact caused by, 6

Ankle, lead placement on, 2–5
Anterior fascicle, anatomy of, 16
APCs. *See* Atrial premature contractions
Artifact
  in atrial premature contraction, 59
  definition of, 6
  from electrical interference, 6
  from movement, 7, 260
  vs pacemaker spike, 228–229
  from poor electrode contact, 8
  in sinus rhythm, 44–45
  vs sinus rhythm with bundle branch block, 261
  in supraventricular tachycardia, 120
  vs ventricular fibrillation, 147
  wandering line as, 8
Atrial depolarization. *See also* PR interval; P wave
  junctional ectopic rhythms in, 115
  representation of
    by PR interval, 25
    by P wave, 14
  retrograde, junctional premature contraction in, 59
Atrial ectopic rhythms. *See also* Atrial fibrillation; Atrial flutter; Atrial tachycardia
  causes of, 98
  rates of, 98
Atrial fibrillation, 110–114, 242–243, 245, 251
  aberration in, 158, 159, 161–162
    vs atrial fibrillation with ventricular tachycardia, 257

Atrial fibrilation, aberration in (*continued*)
    vs atrial fibrillation with ventricular tachycardia, 257
    vs ventricular premature contractions, 169
  vs atrial premature contractions, 255
  vs atrial tachycardia, 123, 246, 255
  with atrioventricular block
    complete, 187–189
      and junctional escape rhythm, *vs* junctional escape rhythm alone, 193
    high grade, 185
  with bundle branch block, 114
    vs ventricular tachycardia, 145–146
  criteria for recognition of, 111
  with dangerous pause, 112
  with multifocal ventricular premature contractions, 113–114
  vs other atrial ectopic rhythms, 120
  with pacemaker, 223
  physiology of, 110–111
  vs sinus tachycardia with bundle branch block, 267
  with ventricular escape beats, 112
  with ventricular premature contraction, 264
  ventricular response to, 111–114
  with ventricular tachycardia, *vs* atrial fibrillation with aberration, 257
  with Wolff–Parkinson–White syndrome, 166
Atrial flutter, 106–110
  aberration in, 158, 159
  vs artifact from muscle movement, 260
  vs atrial fibrillation, 242–243
  with atrioventricular block, high grade, 185
  with 2:1 block
    vs PAT with 2:1 block, 244
    vs sinus rhythm, 263
  with 1:1 conduction, 108
  with 2:1 conduction, 107, 109–110
  criteria for recognition of, 106
  dangers of, 106, 108
  vs junctional tachycardia, 121–122
  vs paroxysmal atrial tachycardia, 123
    with 2:1 block, 253
  physiology of, 106
  rate of, 106
  vs sinus tachycardia, 109
    with bundle branch block, 267
    with first degree AV block and APCs, 256
  with variable block/conduction, 107–109
    vs other atrial ectopic rhythms, 120
  with ventricular premature contractions, *vs* aberration, 168
  ventricular response to, 106–110
Atrial premature contractions, 54–59, 250–251, 269
  aberration in, 159–162
    vs fusion beats, 168

    vs intermittent bundle branch block, 258
    sinus tachycardia with, 249
    vs ventricular inhibited pacemaker, 241
  artifact and, 59
  in bigeminy, 56
    vs PAT with 2:1 block, 124
    sinus bradycardia with, *vs* sinus tachycardia with APC, 69
  criteria for recognition of, 54
  multifocal, atrial tachycardia in, 104
  nonconducted, 57–58, 240
    aberration in, *vs* sinus bradycardia with VPC, 252–253
    vs combination of block types, 252
    vs first and second degree AV block, 246–247
    junctional escape beats and, 81
    vs second degree AV block Mobitz, 192, 243
    vs second degree AV block Wenckebach, 191
    vs sinoatrial block, 208
    vs sinoatrial block with VPCs, 258–259
    vs sinus arrhythmia, 68–69
    ventricular escape beats with, 85
  physiology of, 54
  vs sinus arrhythmia, 68–69
  sinus bradycardia with, 56
  sinus rhythm with, 55–57, 99
    vs atrial fibrillation with VPCs, 264
  sinus tachycardia with, 56–57
  in trigeminy, sinus tachycardia with, *vs* sinus bradycardia with APC, 69
  vs ventricular premature contractions with APCs, 167
Atrial rate, determination of, 36
Atrial repolarization, 14
Atrial tachycardia, 98–101, 246
  with aberrancy, *vs* ventricular tachycardia, 169
  vs atrial fibrillation, 242–243
  with block, *vs* sinus tachycardia with first degree AV block and APCs, 256
  criteria for recognition of, 99
  vs junctional tachycardia, 120
  multifocal, 104–105, 255
    vs atrial fibrillation, 123
    vs atrial premature contractions, 269
    vs atrial tachycardia, 246
    vs other atrial ectopic rhythms, 120
    rate of, 104
    vs sinus tachycardia with first degree AV block and APCs, 256
  paroxysmal
    vs atrial flutter, 123
    with block, 101–103
      and bundle branch block, 102
      criteria for recognition of, 101

INDEX

physiology of, 101
  rate of, 101
with 1:1 block, 99
with 2:1 block, 102–103, 244, 253
  vs nonconducted APCs in bigeminy, 124
  vs sinus rhythm, 263
with 3:1 block, 103
definition of, 98
sinus bradycardia with, 99–100
sinus rhythm with, 99–101
physiology of, 98
rate of, 98
Atrioventricular block, 178–201
  complete, 187–190, 262–263
    atrial fibrillation with, 187
      vs junctional escape rhythm, 193
    vs AV dissociation, 187, 194
    criteria for recognition of, 188
    with junctional escape beats, 268
    with junctional escape rhythm, 190
    physiology of, 187
    with second degree Mobitz block, 247
    vs second degree Wenckebach block, 193, 248–249
    sinus bradycardia with, 188, 190
    vs sinus bradycardia with first degree AV block, 264–265
    ventricular escape rhythm with, 188–190
  definition of, 178
  differential diagnosis of, 191–194
  first degree, 178, 266
    with bundle branch block, sinus rhythm with, 43, 45, 206
    with bundle branch block and second degree SA block Mobitz, 252
    junctional escape beat with, 82
    vs junctional tachycardia, 121
    with nonconducted APC, 58
    vs paroxysmal atrial tachycardia with 2:1 block, 253
    with second degree block and bundle branch block, sinus rhythm with, 243
    with second degree Wenckebach block, 246–247
    sinus bradycardia with, 185, 264–265
    sinus rhythm with, 39, 44, 242
      vs junctional tachycardia, 121
      with ventricular inhibited pacemaker, 241
    with ventricular premature contraction, 66
  high grade, 184–186
    atrial fibrillation with, 185, 245
    atrial flutter with, 185
    criteria for recognition of, 184
    physiology of, 184
    sinus bradycardia with, 185
    sinus rhythm with, 184, 186, 190

    sinus tachycardia with, 186
    with ventricular escape beats, 185–186
  physiology of, 178
  practice ECG strips for, 195–201
  second degree, pacemaker termination of, 222
  second degree Mobitz, 181–183
    bundle branch block with, 266
    vs complete AV block, 247
    criteria for recognition of, 181
    physiology of, 181
    vs second degree Wenckebach block, 192, 246–247
    with second degree Wenckebach block, 182
    sinus bradycardia with, 183, 185
    vs sinus bradycardia
      with first degree AV block, 264–265
      with nonconducted APCs in bigeminy, 192
    vs sinus rhythm, 265
    sinus rhythm with, 181–182
    with VPC, vs sinus bradycardia with VPC, 252–253
  second degree Wenckebach, 178–180
    vs atrial premature contractions, 269
    vs complete AV block, 193, 248–249
    criteria for recognition of, 179
    with first degree block, 246–247
    vs nonconducted APCs, 191
    physiology of, 178
    vs second degree Mobitz block, 192, 246–247
    with second degree Mobitz block, 182
    sinus rhythm with, 179–180, 182
Atrioventricular conduction time, 25. See also PR interval
Atrioventricular dissociation, 115, 118, 259
  vs complete atrioventricular block, 187, 194
  sinus bradycardia with, vs complete atrioventricular block, 268
  in ventricular tachycardia, 138–140
Atrioventricular (AV) node
  anatomy of, 14
  junctional escape beat arising from, 80
  premature contraction at. See Junctional premature contractions
  refractoriness of, in atrial fibrillation, 111
Atrium, anatomy of, 11
AV. See Atrioventricular

Baseline (isoelectric line)
  definition of, 6
  measurement from, 22–23
  wandering, 8
Bigeminy
  in atrial premature contractions, 56
    vs PAT with 2:1 block, 124

INDEX

Bigeminy, in atrial premature contractions (*continued*)
sinus bradycardia with, *vs* sinus tachycardia with
APC in trigeminy, 69
in junctional premature contractions, aberration in,
160
in ventricular premature contractions, 62
in accelerated junctional rhythm, 118
Bipolar leads, definition of, 4
Block, heart. *See* Atrioventricular block; Bundle branch
block; Sinoatrial block
Blood flow in heart, 12
Bradycardia, sinus. *See* Sinus bradycardia
Bundle branch block, 250–251
atrial fibrillation with, 114
vs atrial fibrillation with rapid ventricular response,
251
vs ventricular tachycardia, 145–146
with atrioventricular block
first and second degree, 243
first degree
vs first degree AV block, 242
sinus rhythm with, 43, 45, 206
second degree Mobitz, 266
intermittent, 258
vs premature contractions, 249
junctional tachycardia with, *vs* ventricular tachycardia,
147–148, 248
with paroxysmal atrial tachycardia, 102
rate–related, 41
vs ventricular tachycardia, 148
sinus bradycardia with, 42, 267
sinus rhythm with, 40–41, 119, 206
accelerated idioventricular rhythm after, 137
junctional escape beat in, 81
sinus tachycardia with
vs sinus tachycardia with isolated APC, 250
vs ventricular tachycardia, 145, 149, 254, 259
vs ventricular premature contraction, 70
with ventricular premature contraction, sinus rhythm
with, 67
Bundle branches, anatomy of, 15
Bundle of His, anatomy of, 15

Capture, failure to, by pacemaker, 226–227, 229, 255,
266
Cardiac cells, depolarization/repolarization of, 10. *See
also* Depolarization; Repolarization
Circulation in heart, 12
Conduction in sinus rhythm, 37
Conduction system. *See also* Depolarization; Repolarization
components of, 13–16. *See also specific component*

Delta wave in Wolff–Parkinson–White syndrome, 164–
166
Depolarization. *See also* Atrial depolarization; Ventricular depolarization
definition of, 10
Diaphoresis, wandering baseline in, 8

Ectopic beats. *See* Premature contractions
Ectopic rhythms. *See* Supraventricular ectopic rhythms;
Ventricular ectopic rhythms
Electrical conduction system. *See* Conduction system
Electrical interference, artifact caused by, 6
Electrocardiogram, definition of, 2
Electrodes. *See also* Leads
loose, ventricular fibrillation simulated by, 147
placement of, 2–3
poor contact of, artifact caused by, 8
Electrophysiology. *See* Conduction system; Depolarization; Repolarization
End diastolic ventricular premature contractions. *See
under* Ventricular premature contractions
Escape beats
definition of, 80
differential diagnosis of, 87–88
junctional. *See* Junctional escape beats
practice ECG strips for, 89–95
ventricular. *See* Ventricular escape beats
Escape rhythms
junctional, 83, 189–190, 261
practice ECG strips for, 89–95
ventricular, 86, 189–190
Extrasystoles. *See* Premature contractions

Failure to capture by pacemaker, 226–227, 229, 255,
266
Failure to sense by pacemaker, 224–225, 229, 255–266
Fascicles, anatomy of, 16
Fibrillation. *See* Atrial fibrillation; Ventricular fibrillation
Fibrillatory (f) wave, 110–114
Flutter. *See* Atrial flutter; Ventricular flutter
Fusion beats, 64
vs atrial premature contractions with aberrancy, 168
f (fibrillatory) wave, 110–114
F (flutter) wave, 106–110

Graph paper, measurements on
practice ECG strips for, 29–33
PR interval, 25, 27
QRS interval, 26, 28
time, 24
voltage, 22–23

INDEX

Heart
  anatomy of, 11–12
  blood flow in, 12
Heart rate
  determination of, 36
  in sinus rhythm, 37
His, bundle of, anatomy of, 15

Idioventricular rhythm, accelerated, 136–137
Inhibited pacemaker mode, 221–223
Interatrial septum, anatomy of, 11
Internodal pathways, anatomy of, 13
Interpolated ventricular premature contractions, 65
Intervals. *See also specific interval*
  types of, 20
Interventricular septum, anatomy of, 11
Isoelectric line (baseline). *See* Baseline

JPCs. *See* Junctional premature contractions
Junctional ectopic rhythms, 115–119. *See also Junc-
    tional tachycardia*
  accelerated, 245
    after sinus rhythm with bundle branch block, 119
    atrioventricular dissociation and, 118
    criteria for recognition of, 116
    physiology of, 115
    P waves in, 116–119
    rate of, 115
    with ventricular premature contractions, 118
  atrioventricular dissociation and, 115, 118
  with bundle branch block, 119
  criteria for recognition of, 116
  physiology of, 115
  P waves in, 116–119
  rates of, 115
  with ventricular premature contractions, 117–118
Junctional escape beats, 80–82
  after malignant ventricular premature contraction, 117
  atrial premature contractions and, 81
  criteria for recognition of, 80
  vs junctional premature contractions, 88
  physiology of, 80
  sinus rhythm with, 81–82
  ventricular premature contractions with, 81–82
Junctional escape rhythms, 83
  vs atrial fibrillation with complete AV block and junc-
      tional escape rhythm, 193
  with atrial standstill, 261
  in complete atrioventricular block, 189–190
Junctional premature contractions, 59–62

aberration in, 159–160
  criteria for recognition of, 60
  junctional ectopic rhythms and, 115
  vs junctional escape beats, 88
  nonconducted, 60
  physiology of, 59
  sinus bradycardia with, 61
  sinus rhythm with, 61–62
    ventricular escape beats with, 85
  trigeminy pattern of, 61
  vs ventricular premature contractions, 267
Junctional tachycardia
  aberration in, 163
  vs atrial fibrillation, 242–243
  vs atrial flutter, 121–122*
  vs atrial tachycardia, 120
  with bundle branch block, *vs* ventricular tachycardia,
      147–148, 248
  criteria for recognition of, 116
  vs paroxysmal atrial tachycardia with 2:1 block, 244
  physiology of, 115
  P waves in, 117, 119
  rate of, 115
  vs sinus rhythm with first degree AV block, 121
  with ventricular premature contractions, 117

Lead I, description of, 4
Lead II, description of, 4
Lead III, description of, 5
Leads. *See also* Electrodes
  bipolar, definition of, 4
  placement of, 2–3
  standard, 4–5
Left anterior fascicle, anatomy of, 16
Left bundle branch, anatomy of, 15
Left posterior fascicle, anatomy of, 16

Malignant ventricular premature contractions, 65, 67,
    117
Measurements. *See* Graph paper, measurements on
Mobitz block. *See under* Atrioventricular block; Sino-
    atrial block
Movement, artifact caused by, 7, 260
Multifocal atrial tachycardia. *See under* Atrial tachycar-
    dia
Multifocal ventricular premature contractions. *See under*
    Ventricular premature contractions
Muscle tremor, artifact caused by, 7
Myocardial infarction, wandering baseline in, 8

Nodal premature contractions (NPCs). *See* Junctional premature contractions

One–lead monitoring, 2–8
  artifacts in, 6–8
  definition of, 2
  in emergency situations, 5
  lead placement in, 2–3
  standard leads for, 4–5
Oxygenation of blood, 12

Pacemaker (mechanical), 220–237
  capture by, 220
  definition of, 220
  differential diagnosis with, 228–230
  in inhibited mode, normal function of, 221–223
  malfunction of
    vs artifact from muscle movement, 260
    failure to capture, 226–227
    failure to sense, 224–225
      vs failure to capture, 229, 255, 266
    normal function of, 220–223
      vs malfunction, 230
    practice ECG strips for, 231–237
  programmable, 223
  spike of, 220
    vs artifact, 228–229
    atrial *vs* ventricular, 220
    in failure to capture, 226–227
    in failure to sense, 224–225
  in triggered mode, normal function of, 221
Paper for electrocardiogram. *See* Graph paper
Paroxysmal atrial tachycardia (PAT). *See under* Atrial tachycardia
Polarization. *See* Depolarization; Repolarization
Posterior fascicle, anatomy of, 16
P–P cycle
  in heart rate determination, 36
  in sinoatrial block, 204–207
  in sinus arrhythmia, 42
  in sinus bradycardia with bundle branch block, 42
  in sinus rhythm, 41
    with first degree AV block and bundle branch block, 43
  in sinus tachycardia, 42
Premature contractions, 54–77
  atrial. *See* Atrial premature contractions
  AV nodal (junctional). *See* Junctional premature contractions

differential diagnosis of, 68–70
measurement of, practice ECG strips for, 71–77
supraventricular, 54
types of, 54
ventricular. *See* Ventricular premature contractions
PR interval
  in atrial tachycardia, 104–105
  in atrioventricular block
    complete, 187–190
    first degree, 39
    high grade, 184
    second degree Mobitz, 181–183
    second degree Wenckebach, 178–180
  definition of, 20
  in junctional escape beat, 80, 82
  measurement of, 25, 27
    in emergency, 26–27
    practice ECG strips for, 29–33
  normal range for, 25
  in sinus tachycardia with accelerated AV conduction, 40
  in Wolff–Parkinson–White syndrome, 164–166
PR segment, definition of, 20
Purkinje fibers, anatomy of, 16
P wave
  in aberration, 158–159, 161–163
  in accelerated idioventricular rhythm, 136–137
  in atrial premature contraction, 54–58
  in atrial tachycardia, 98–100
    multifocal, 104–105
    paroxysmal, with block, 101–103
  in atrioventricular block, 178
    complete, 187–188
    high grade, 184
    second degree Mobitz, 181–183
    second degree Wenckebach, 178–180
  definition of, 14
  in junctional ectopic rhythms, 115–119
  in junctional escape beat, 80–82
  in junctional escape rhythm, 83
  in junctional premature contraction, 59–62
  pacemaker inhibition by, 222
  replacement of
    in atrial fibrillation, 111
    by flutter wave, 106
  in sinoatrial block, 204–205
  in ventricular premature contraction, 64, 66–67
  in ventricular tachycardia, 139–140

QRS complex
  in accelerated idioventricular rhythm, 136–137
  in atrial fibrillation, 111

in atrial flutter, 106–107
in atrial premature contraction, 54, 57–58
in atrial tachycardia, 99–100
   multifocal, 104
   paroxysmal, block, 101–103
in atrioventricular block
   complete, 187–189
   second degree Wenckebach, 179
components of, 17
in junctional ectopic rhythms, 115–116
in junctional escape beat, 80, 82
in junctional premature contraction, 59–60
in normal mechanically paced function, 220–221
in pacemaker failure to capture, 226–227
in pacemaker failure to sense, 225
in sinoatrial block, 204–205
in sinus rhythm with bundle branch block, 40–41
temporary variation of. *See* Aberration
types of, 18
in ventricular escape beat, 84
in ventricular fibrillation, 143, 145–149
in ventricular flutter, 141
in ventricular premature contraction, 62, 64, 66–67,
   70
in ventricular tachycardia, 138–139
in Wolff–Parkinson–White syndrome, 164–166
QRS interval
   measurement of, 26, 28
      practice ECG strips for, 29–33
   normal range for, 26
QT interval, definition of, 20
Q wave
   measurement of, 22
   negative deflection of, 17–18

Refractory period, definition of, 10
Relative refractory period, 10
Repolarization. *See also* Atrial repolarization; Ventricular
   repolarization
   definition of, 10
Right bundle branch, anatomy of, 15
R–R cycle
   in atrial fibrillation, 111–113
   in heart rate determination, 36
   in sinus arrhythmia, 42
   in sinus bradycardia with bundle branch block, 42
   in sinus rhythm, 41
      with first degree AV block and bundle branch
        block, 43
   in sinus tachycardia, 42
R wave
   measurement of, 22

positive deflection of, 17–18
R' wave, description of, 18

SA. *See* Sinoatrial
Segments. *See also specific segment*
   types of, 20
Sense, failure to, by pacemaker, 224–225, 229, 255,
   266
Septum
   interatrial, anatomy of, 11
   interventricular, anatomy of, 11
Sinoatrial block, 204–217
   vs atrial premature contractions, 250–251
      nonconducted, 208, 240
   differential diagnosis of, 208–210
   first degree, 204
   pacemaker termination of, 222
   practice ECG strips for, 211–217
   second degree Mobitz, 204–207
      with bundle branch block, 252
      criteria for recognition of, 205
      physiology of, 204
   second degree Wenckebach
      criteria for recognition of, 204
      physiology of, 204
   vs sinus arrhythmia, 209–210, 256–257
   sinus bradycardia with, 207
   with ventricular premature contractions, *vs* noncon-
      ducted APCs, 258–259
Sinoatrial node (SA node, sinus node), anatomy of, 13
   failure of, junctional escape rhythms in, 83
Sinus arrest. *See* Sinoatrial block
Sinus arrhythmia, 39, 42
   vs atrial premature contractions, 68–69, 240
   vs combination of block types, 252
   definition of, 37
   vs sinoatrial block, 209–210, 256–257
   types of, 37–38
Sinus bradycardia
   accelerated idioventricular rhythm after, 137
   atrial premature contractions with, 56
      aberrant, 162
   atrial tachycardia with, 99–100
   with atrioventricular block, 185, 190
      first degree, 264–265
      first degree and second degree Mobitz, 183
   with AV dissociation, *vs* complete AV block, 268
   with bundle branch block, 42, 267
   definition of, 37–38
   with junctional premature contractions, 61
   with sinoatrial block, 207
   with supraventricular tachycardia, aberrant, 161

Sinus bradycardia (*continued*)
  ventricular escape beat with, 85
  with ventricular premature contraction, 252–253
    and APC, *vs* sinus bradycardia with VPC, 252–253
Sinus node. *See* Sinoatrial node
Sinus rhythm
  with atrial premature contractions, 55–57
    aberrant, 161
    junctional escape beats and VPC with, 81
  with atrial premature contractions and VPCs, *vs* atrial
    fibrillation with VPC, 264
  with atrial tachycardia, 99–101
  with atrioventricular block. *See under* Atrioventricular
    block
  with bundle branch block. *See under* Bundle branch
    block
  conduction in, 37
  definition of, 37
  with intermittent Wolff–Parkinson–White syndrome,
    166
  with junctional escape beats, 81–82
  with junctional premature contractions, 61–62
    and ventricular escape beats, 85
  measurement of, artifact in, 44–45
  normal, 37 *vs* second degree AV block Mobitz, 265
  with sinoatrial block, 206
  vs tachycardia, 263
  with ventricular premature contractions, 62–67
    and ventricular escape beats, 85
  with ventricular tachycardia, 139–141
Sinus tachycardia, 42, 250
  with accelerated AV conduction, 40
  artifact in, 44
  vs atrial flutter, 109
  with atrial premature contractions, 56–57
    aberrant, 249
    vs sinus tachycardia with first degree AV block and
      APCs, 256
  with atrial premature contractions in trigeminy, *vs* si-
    nus bradycardia with APC in bigeminy, 69
  with atrioventricular block
    complete, 188
    first degree and APCs, 256
      vs PAT with 2:1 block, 253
    high grade, 186
  with bundle branch block, *vs* ventricular tachycardia,
    145, 149, 254, 259
  definition of, 37–38
  with ventricular premature contractions, 67
Spike of pacemaker. *See under* Pacemaker (mechanical)
ST depression, measurement of, 23
ST elevation, measurement of, 23

ST segment
  definition of, 20
  in ventricular flutter, 141
Supraventricular beats, definition of, 54
Supraventricular ectopic rhythms. *See also* Atrial ec-
    topic rhythms; Junctional ectopic rhythms
  differential diagnosis of, 121–124
  practice ECG strips for, 125–133
  tachycardia, 120
Supraventricular premature beats, 250–251
  aberrant, *vs* ventricular premature contractions, 167
Supraventricular tachycardia, 54, 120, 262
  aberration in, 162
  with bundle branch block or aberration, *vs* ventricular
    tachycardia, 254
  in Wolff–Parkinson–White syndrome, 164–165
S wave
  measurement of, 22
  negative deflection of, 17–18
S' wave, description of, 18
Sweating, wandering baseline in, 8

Tachycardia. *See also* Atrial tachycardia; Junctional
    tachycardia; Sinus tachycardia; Supraventricu-
    lar tachycardia
Ta wave, 14
Time, measurement of, on graph paper, 24
Torso, lead placement on, 2–3
Tremor, artifact caused by, 7
Trigeminy
  in atrial premature contractions, 269
    sinus tachycardia with, *vs* sinus bradycardia with
      APC in bigeminy, 69
  in junctional premature contractions, 61
Triggered pacemaker mode, 221
T wave
  in atrial premature contractions, 55, 57–58
  description of, 19
  in ventricular flutter, 141

Unifocal ventricular premature contractions, 63–67
U wave, description of, 19

Ventricle(s)
  anatomy of, 11
  conduction system of, 15–16
  response of
    in atrial fibrillation, 111–114
    to atrial flutter, 106–110
Ventricular depolarization. *See also* QRS complex; QRS
    interval

accelerated idioventricular rhythm in, 136
representation of
by QRS complex, 17–18
by QRS interval, 26
ventricular tachycardia in, 138
in Wolff–Parkinson–White syndrome, 164
Ventricular ectopic rhythms, 136–156
accelerated idioventricular rhythm, 136–137
causes of, 136
differential diagnosis of, 145–149
practice ECG strips for, 150–156
rates of, 136
ventricular fibrillation, 140, 143–144, 147
ventricular flutter, 141–142
ventricular tachycardia. *See* Ventricular tachycardia
Ventricular escape beats
with atrial fibrillation, 112
with atrial premature contractions, 85
criteria for recognition of, 84
with high grade atrioventricular block, 185–186
physiology of, 84
sinus bradycardia with, 84–85
sinus rhythm with, 85
vs ventricular premature contractions, 87
with ventricular premature contractions, 84–85
vs ventricular inhibited pacemaker, 241
Ventricular escape rhythms, 86
in complete atrioventricular block, 188–190
Ventricular fibrillation, 143–144
vs artifact, 147
ventricular tachycardia progressing to, 140
Ventricular flutter, 141–142
Ventricular inhibited pacemaker, 241
malfunction of, 224–227
normal function of, 221–223
Ventricular premature contractions, 62–67
vs aberration, 158
vs atrial fibrillation with aberration, 169
atrial flutter with, *vs* aberration, 168
vs atrial premature contractions, 250–251
with atrial premature contractions, *vs* all APCs,
167
vs atrial premature contractions with aberration,
249
atrioventricular block and APC with, 66
in bigeminy, 62
accelerated junctional rhythm with, 118
bundle branch block with, 67
criteria for recognition of, 66
end diastolic, 64, 67
vs bundle branch block, 70
vs ventricular escape beats, 87
vs intermittent bundle branch block, 258
interpolated, 65

junctional escape beats and, 81–82
vs junctional premature contractions, 267
malignant, 65, 67
junctional tachycardia with, 117
multifocal, 63
with atrial fibrillation, 113–114
junctional tachycardia with, 117
with pacemaker beat, 241
pacemaker inhibition by, 222
physiology of, 62
sinus bradycardia with, 252–253
sinus tachycardia with, 67
vs supraventricular premature beat with aberration,
167
trigeminy pattern of, 63
unifocal, 63–67
with ventricular escape beats, 84–85
vs ventricular inhibited pacemaker, 241
ventricular tachycardia caused by, 138, 139
Ventricular rate, determination of, 36
Ventricular repolarization, 19. *See also* T wave
Ventricular tachycardia, 138–141
vs aberration, 158
vs atrial fibrillation, 251
with bundle branch block, 145–146
vs atrial tachycardia with aberration, 169
atrioventricular dissociation with, 140
criteria for recognition of, 139
vs junctional tachycardia with bundle branch block,
147–148, 248
physiology of, 138
progressing to ventricular fibrillation, 140
vs rate–related bundle branch block, 148
sinus rhythm with, 139–141
vs sinus tachycardia, 250
with bundle branch block, 145, 149, 254, 259
vs supraventricular tachycardia with bundle branch
block, 254
Voltage, measurement of, on graph paper, 22–23
VPCs. *See* Ventricular premature contractions

Wandering baseline, 8
Wenckebach block. *See under* Atrioventricular block;
Sinoatrial block
Wolff–Parkinson–White syndrome, 164–166
with atrial fibrillation, 166
criteria for recognition of, 165
delta waves in, 164–166
intermittent, 166
physiology of, 164
supraventricular tachycardia and, 164
Wrist, lead placement on, 2–5